# Catering Questions & Answers: Food Hygiene

**Geoff Ward**



CRONER CCH

Croner.CCH Group Limited
145 London Road
Kingston upon Thames
Surrey KT2 6SR
Tel: 020 8547 3333

Published by
Croner.CCH Group Limited
145 London Road
Kingston upon Thames
Surrey KT2 6SR
Tel: 020 8547 3333

First published January 1995
Second Edition 1998
Third Edition 2000



British Library cataloguing in Publication Data. A CIP Catalogue Record for this book is available from the British Library

ISBN 1 85524 552 3

Printed by Creative Print and Design, Wales

# AUTHOR

**GEOFF WARD,** TD, MCIEH, MRSH, MIOSH, FRSTM&H, MWM Soc, Geoff is a highly respected Environmental Health Officer with over 26 years active involvement in the profession. He has committed his life to innovation in the public health arena. He has drawn on his life experience in military, local government and commercial fields to innovate and develop simple systems for complex problems.

Geoff started his environmental health career in 1974 within H M Forces by joining the Royal Army Medical Corps from school at the age of 18 years. He was trained as a hygiene assistant and developed a keen interest in preventative health disciplines and tropical medicine.
In 1977 he left H M Forces with a view to accelerating his career by joining local government. His first post was as a pest control officer for the City of Manchester. Switching to the role of drainage examiner, within the year he had secured a place on the student environmental health officers' programme and studied for his Diploma in Environmental Health at Salford College. He qualified in 1981 and was elected to the Chartered Institute of Environmental Health. Geoff was then appointed district EHO for two of the toughest areas of the city — Hulme and Mosside — a real testing ground for a first appointment! He successfully studied for the Diploma in air pollution control the following year and was elected to the Royal Society for the promotion of health. In 1981 and 1982 Geoff undertook a public health study tour of India and also, as an independent traveller, made the overland journey to Pakistan. These adventures laid the foundation for UK encouragement of EHOs to share their public health experience overseas and led to the establishment of the International Federation of Environmental Health. Geoff served, in all, seven years at Manchester and held subsequent posts of default works branch officer (housing repair and abatement of public health nuisances in default of notices) and also specialist EHO city centre.

He entered the commercial world of environmental health by securing the post of food hygiene and safety consultant south west for Forte Hotels (formally Trusthouse Forte). He moved to the Bath area in 1984 to take up this appointment and gained considerable practical experience in the implementation of food safety and health and safety management systems within every aspect of the group's operation: — hotels, commercial, in-store, airports and roadside catering, also food manufacturing and distribution. He worked for the well established group food services department and assisted in the development of policy concepts, training and also managed the control of the first large viral gastroenteritis outbreaks in the mid-1980s with some considerable degree of success.

In 1988 Geoff left Forte to establish his own environmental health consultancy business Hygiene Monitoring Services Ltd. This initially focused on the hotel and catering industry and quickly established a reputation for simple solutions to complex new legal requirements from highly motivational training and a client focused approach. Geoff took on good staff early in the business history who he motivated to drive forward, gaining many blue chip clients including P&O courses, Cadbury Ltd, Accor Group Hotels, ASDA, Airtours to name a few. The business was incorporated to form a limited company in 1993 and moved to its present location with offices and a training suite based in Bath. He was the first to develop the concept of the "company food safety policy" in order for organisations to establish the "due diligence" defence under the **Food Safety Act 1990**. Geoff was a semi-finalist in the Business Person of the Year HTV West in 1991 and also in 1992. He achieved a National Training Award Regional Winner in 1993.

He is now managing director of HMS Ltd which employs 24 staff throughout the UK. He has established a strong management team, which now runs all the operational activities of the business. Geoff remains at the head of the organisation and is a regular speaker at national and international seminars and conferences on food and safety issues. He is keen to spread the message of learning lessons from the past and using best practice to achieve the highest control of these potential business threats. He has had a clear focus of supporting industry with its efforts to achieve compliance with national statutes. Geoff continues to maintain his active involvement within the profession through the Chartered Institute of Environmental Health, supporting both local and national activities. He is a keen advocate of the mentoring of student EHOs and has supported the University of the West of England with a placement scheme at HMS which has successfully run for the past 5 years, putting back into the profession some fine and able EHOs. He has maintained his links with the Forces, having now served for 26 years achieving the rank of Major in the Territorial Army.

# Acknowledgement

Geoff would like to acknowledge the encouragement, help and support from the consultants and administrators at Hygiene Monitoring Services Ltd. Everyone is so busy these days but they all found time for Geoff to gain another prospective on the many questions, which are commonly asked, and contained in this book.

# THE REVIEWER

**MICHAEL J BOELLA,** MA,
is principal lecturer at the University of Brighton Business School and editor of Croner's *Catering*. He is the author of Human Resource Management in the Hospitality Industry, published by Stanley Thornes. He worked previously with Forte and Co Ltd, Bass and Price Waterhouse.

# THE FOOD CHAIN

## THE FOOD PRODUCTION CHAIN

### The Food Protection Chain

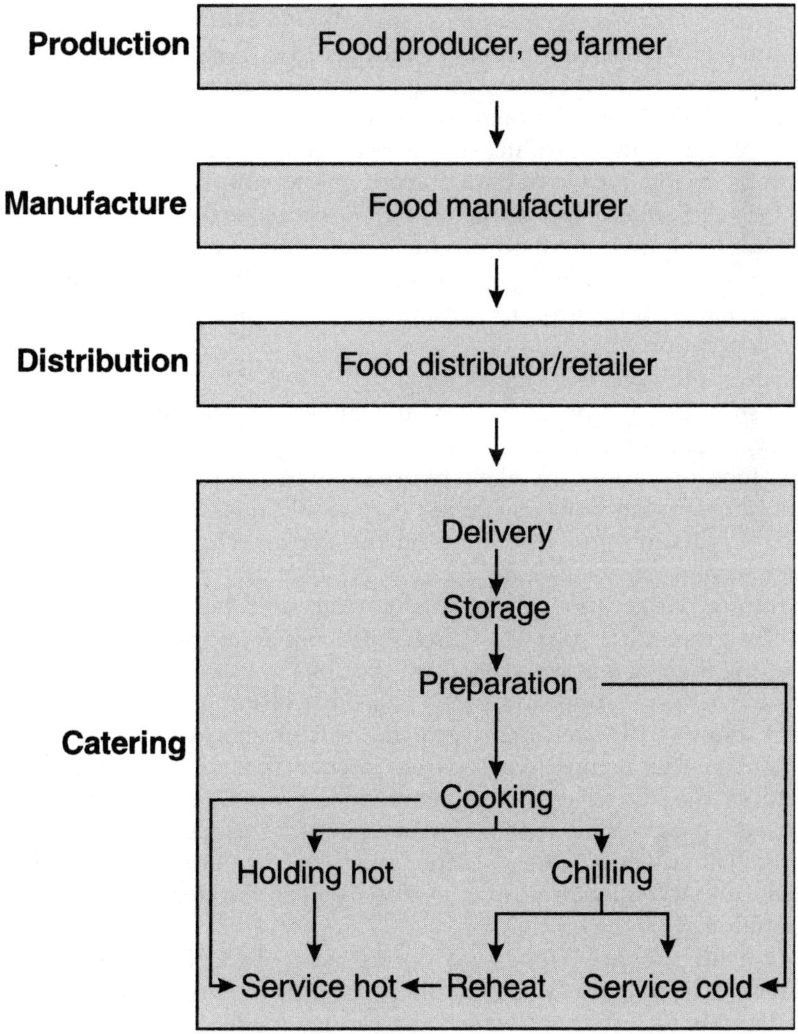

Food producers and manufacturers range from local small-scale family operations, eg bakers, pie makers, and producers of cooked meats, cheese and pâté, to the large international companies producing frozen foods, canned products, coffee, chocolate and dry mixes and flour millers. They might have their own distribution networks from depots around the UK but many supply wholesale distributors from which caterers can obtain a large range of products and which simplify ordering and payment procedures, with generous discounts for bulk purchase. These companies may specialise in particular lines such as frozen ready meals or general dry produce. Some may have a vast range of "across the board" products, making deliveries perhaps six or seven days a week. There is a rapid move toward duel delivery, where meat, vegetable and other product suppliers team up to gain the transport cost savings. Many suppliers though, continue to supply particular market niches, eg fish and chip trade or high-street bakers.

Once supplied, the food products pass along four main routes:

- dry goods — to the dry goods store, often called ambient goods
- vegetables and grocery products — to the vegetable store or refrigeration
- frozen produce — to the freezer
- fresh perishable products — to the chillers or cold rooms.

The type of operation dictates the relative proportions of these products. Fast-food operations are likely to use more frozen products and limited amounts of salad type vegetables; they would therefore have little need for refrigeration and rely more on the freezer. High-class restaurants may have a great need for fresh vegetables and perishable products requiring refrigeration, eg fresh fish, meats and dairy products.

The preparation phase is essentially similar in most businesses. In catering there is a move away from the days of in-house butcheries and bakeries. Even "spud and other vegetable bashing" has been dealt a fatal blow with the ready-peeled, vacuum-packed products now available. This is most useful when kitchen space is limited and often reduces the risk of cross-contamination. Frozen ready meals, cakes, gateaux, etc also play a part in many catering businesses where speedy consistent quality and a wide range of products is a priority. Vacuum-packed meats play an essential role in the steakhouse pub-type operation.

Not all prepared foods go on to be cooked. Confectionery and patisserie products, salads, sandwiches prepared from cooked meats and/or cheeses pass straight to the service mode. Some cooked foods may be chilled and assembled for buffet or used in the preparation of foods to be served cold. Cooking is the last hope for destruction of harmful micro-organisms. Only quick cooling and refrigeration will prevent food poisoning from spore-forming bacteria. Undercooking may leave harmful bacteria alive, such as Salmonella species, or perhaps only serve to incubate the bacteria inherent in most raw foods.

The service mode can be quite diverse depending on the sector of the catering market. For schools and hospital catering, foods may be transferred from a central production unit, hot or chilled, and served or re-heated at its final destination. In the restaurant and hotel catering business the aim should be to produce all hot food fresh from the oven but nevertheless a vast amount of preparation (cook chill) is done in advance. In these days of tight margins, strict cost controls in terms of staffing, food costs and high property costs, there is a need to balance quality against these costs without compromising food hygiene. These are the essential issues for business proprietors and managers particularly when considering the need to define and implement the legal requirement to do hazard analysis — within *all* food businesses.

# CATERING QUESTIONS & ANSWERS: FOOD HYGIENE

## FOOD SOURCES AND MANUFACTURING

Q1 What potential micro-organisms could be present on meat and what are their origins?

Q2 How can I tell if red meat is fit to eat?

Q3 How can I tell if frozen red meat is fit to eat?

Q4 How can I tell if vaccum-packed red meat is fit to eat?

Q5 Why is raw poultry contaminated with Salmonella?

Q6 Are there any other conditions which may affect poultry that the caterer should be aware of?

Q7 How can I tell if poultry meat is fit?

Q8 What is the likelihood of my eggs being contaminated by Salmonella and causing food poisoning?

Q9 Are free-range eggs better than battery-farm eggs?

Q10 What are the alternatives to using fresh-shell eggs?

Q11 Is it safe to drink raw milk and cream?

Q12 How is milk heat-treated?

Q13 Why does pasteurised milk still have a limited shelf-life even within a refrigerator?

Q14 With so many cheeses available how can I assess the fitness and safety of cheese?

Q15 I have heard much about soft cheeses being contaminated by Listeria organisms. How does this occur and how can the infection be prevented?

Q16 How can I ensure the quality and freshness of fruit and vegetables for my catering operation?

Q17 What causes fruit and vegetables to spoil?

Q18 Are organic foods more safe than the mass-produced foods?

Q19 There has been much in the news about E.coli 0157. Is this a new organism and where does it come from?

Q20 What are the implications of the dioxin contamination of food during the 1999 Belgian food incident?

## VEGETARIAN FOODS

Q21 What are the main bacterial risks with vegetarian catering, considering that meat, poultry and fish are not used?

Q22 Why is it necessary to pre-soak dry pulses prior to cooking?

## FOOD PRESERVATION

Q23 Are there any risks from the use and consumption of irradiated foods?

Q24 Should I always purchase foods which do not contain additives?

Q25 What can the caterer do to extend the life of food?

Q26 Why is vacuum-packing hazardous?

Q27 Why should I use preserved foods when so much fresh food is available?

Q28 What is meant by "ambient temperature" and how can convenience foods be preserved so they can be stored at such temperatures?

## GENETICALLY MODIFIED FOODS

Q29 What are genetically modified foods and can they be harmful to health?

Q30 How can I best ensure I am not being supplied with food that has genetically modified ingredients?

Q31 What training should be given to my staff about genetically modified foods?

Q32 What genetically modified foods are approved for human consumption?

Q33 What are my legal obligations with respect to labelling of menu items containing genetically modified foods?

Q34 How are GM foods approved for safety?

## FOOD SUPPLY

Q35 What should I check if I carry out a "due diligence" audit of one of my suppliers?

Q36 I do not feel experienced enough to do my company's supplier audits. What are my options?

Q37 What should I check when receiving deliveries?

Q38 How often should I have food delivered for my catering operation?

Q39 What shall I do if one of my suppliers is prosecuted for hygiene offences?

Q40 What should I do if I receive a complaint from a customer that I believe to be a supplier problem?

Q41 The concept of due diligence appears to require my organisation to audit our suppliers and it occurs to me that all other organisations are doing a similar task. Why can we not pool our meagre resources and have all suppliers audited and approved centrally rather than carrying out so many visits individually?

Q42 Is the purchase of pre-prepared and pre-packed raw meats and vegetables a safer and more hygienic option than on-site preparation in the kitchen and, if so, is the increased cost a fair reflection of the contamination/food poisoning risks avoided?

## FOOD STORAGE

Q43 How can I get the best from my food storage facilities?

Q44 What is "freezer burn"?

Q45 Why can refrigerated foods be stored quite legally at 8°C when clearly this is in the danger zone?

Q46 I notice small flies in my vegetable storage area. What are they and how can I get rid of them?

Q47 What foods need to be stored under refrigeration?

Q48 What are the rules on storing boxes within freezers and refrigerators?

Q49 I have heard the term "double stacking" mentioned with respect to refrigerators. What does it mean and how can I prevent it?

Q50 What should I do if a freezer breaks down?

Q51 How often should I defrost my chest freezers?

Q52 How often should I check the temperature of my refrigerators?

Q53 How long will food last under refrigeration and within freezers?

Q54 Is there any value in labelling refrigerators and shelving to ensure risks of cross-contamination are prevented?

Q55 With all the publicity regarding E.coli 0157 in meat, do I now have to keep raw meat separate from cooked products?

Q56 I have limited space within my dry store. Why do I have to keep food off the floor?

Q57 I have only a limited dry store facility which is a long way from the kitchen. Why can I not use the kitchen for day-to-day dry storage?

Q58 Where should I store eggs?

Q59 What temperature should ice cream be kept at if I wish to scoop it straight from the tub?

Q60 How can I tell the freshness of shellfish supplies?

Q61 How can I tell the freshness of crabs and lobsters?

Q62 How should I store fresh fish?

Q63 What is the best method of storing poultry to prevent risk of contamination?

Q64 If I purchase a bought-in wrapped meat pie with a "use by" date on the product and I do not use it or sell it, can I freeze it for sale on another occasion, providing I do so before the "use by" date?

Q65 What is the difference between yoghurts which can be stored at room temperature and those which have to be refrigerated?

## PERSONAL HYGIENE

Q66 How long does a person remain infectious after having suffered from food poisoning?

Q67 What is the most common source of infection from a food handler?

Q68 What risk is there from wearing normal clothing while handling food?

Q69 Why should head coverings be worn in a food area?

Q70 Why should I not smoke in and around food rooms and can I smoke a pipe?

Q71 Is there a definitive list of when staff should wash their hands?

Q72 What is the best form of hand-drying facility for a catering unit?

Q73 Is there any food safety advantage to my staff wearing disposable gloves while handling high-risk foods?

Q74 When do food handlers have to report infections?

Q75 Is it necessary to provide hand-washing facilities at temporary outdoor barbecues?

## PESTS

Q76 I have a problem with flies within my catering business. What are the practical solutions?

Q77 Where are electronic fly-killing units best sited?

Q78 Are electronic fly-killing units a necessary requirement in all food areas?

Q79 A number of my customers have noticed small black flies hovering around the bar areas. What are they and how may they be eliminated?

Q80 Can a cockroach infestation be fully eliminated from a food premises?

Q81 I believe that my outside areas are infested with rats. What are the most common signs of infestation and possible sources?

Q82 I believe my pest control operator is feeding the rodents rather than trying to get rid of them. What should I do? The infestation persists.

Q83 What sort of poisons are available for killing rodents and can I carry out the work myself?

Q84 I have noticed a rather horrible odour in and around the public rooms in my unit. What is it likely to be and what is the solution?

Q85 What is the difference between food pest and incidental pest?

Q86 How can I get rid of birds from my kitchen?

Q87 My EHO has requested that I fit fly screens to all my kitchen windows. Do I really have to go to the expense?

Q88 My EHO has said that all the waste bins in my kitchen must be kept lidded. Is this really a practical proposition when they are constantly in use throughout the day?

## CATERING DESIGN

Q89 What are the most important aspects of design for a kitchen?

Q90 What are good tips to ensure my kitchen can be easily and effectively cleaned?

Q91 I am considering a new floor for my kitchen. What is the best surface recommended?

Q92 How can I ensure that the requirements for floors are met when they have to be non-slip surfaces for health and safety purposes, yet cleansable with respect to food hygiene?

Q93 I have been recommended to have a grease trap installed within the catering area. Will this cause problems?

Q94 Whatever happened to kitchen drains? We seemed so much better off with them.

## FOOD PREPARATION

Q95 Why are wooden utensils and cutting boards no longer satisfactory for food handling? I have heard that polypropylene scratches easily and contains more bacteria than wood.

Q96 How can I prevent cross-contamination within my kitchen?

Q97 Why is the cooling of food so vitally important to food hygiene?

Q98 Does all food have to be defrosted before it is cooked?

Q99 My refrigerator is a long way from the hot kitchen. How long can I keep raw meat and fish out before it must be cooked?

Q100 Why should pot plants not be allowed in food preparation or service areas?

Q101 How can I ensure the safe washing of fruits and salad items so that they are ready for consumption by the consumer?

Q102 Can sanitisers be used for washing salad and fruit items as well as to disinfect food contact surfaces?

Q103 What special precautions do I have to undertake when carrying out catering outdoors?

Q104 Why do some pre-prepared sandwiches have a lot of information on the packaging while others have none? As a caterer, do I have to label the sandwiches that I prepare?

## COOKING AND REHEATING

Q105 What are the main hazards in using a microwave for cooking and how can I overcome them?

Q106 Without using a probe thermometer how can I tell if food is thoroughly cooked?

Q107 Why is there a need to cook burgers thoroughly when beef can be eaten rare?

Q108 Is there any health risk in producing rare beef and steaks for my customers?

Q109 I often cook joints of meat on one day, then cool them down and reheat the next day. How long can I hold each food and to what temperature should I reheat it?

Q110 What is the difference between the core temperature of food when it is cooked and the holding temperature of food during service? Why is there such a difference?

Q111 Can I be sure that reheating pre-cooked food will make it safe if it has been at room temperature for a while?

Q112 What are the main foreign material risks within the kitchen?

Q113 How can risks from foreign matter be reduced?

Q114 I have heard much about keeping food reasonably cool while it is being prepared. What advice is there to ensure this is undertaken?

Q115 Does blast chilling have a role to play in small catering establishments or is it merely a high-volume mass production tool?

Q116 I am considering purchasing a vacuum-packing machine for my catering business as I understand the life of foods can be made considerably longer. Are there any risks from using such equipment?

Q117 How can I ensure that chickens and other poultry are thoroughly cooked before service?

Q118 Is there any advantage in using the self-sanitising "Microban" cutting boards?

Q119 How can I ensure E.coli 0157 is prevented in my kitchen?

## CLEANING

Q120 How many cleaning products do I need for an average kitchen?

Q121 What is the difference between sanitisers and disinfectants and when should they be used?

Q122 What is the best, most effective sanitising agent for my kitchens?

Q123 Why are my detergents not successful against all grease and dirt found within the kitchen?

Q124 A black line has built up around the edges of the toilet accommodation, bars and areas of the kitchen. Why does this occur and how can it be prevented?

Q125 Are mops and buckets the most satisfactory method of floor cleaning within kitchen areas?

Q126 Is there any alternative to the mop and bucket for cleaning floors?

Q127 What is the best method of ensuring sanitisation of food contact surfaces within kitchens?

Q128 How can I ensure that my sanitisers for food contact surfaces remain of adequate strength for their period of use?

Q129 I do not have a dishwasher in my small catering unit. What is the best method of cleaning crockery?

Q130 I have problems with waste food in that nobody seems to wish to collect it these days. What is the best solution to this disposal problem?

Q131 I am aware that chlorine-based chemical sanitisers affect aluminium and anodised surfaces, including shelving and meat slicers. How can I ensure adequate sanitisation of such equipment?

Q132 What is the best method of ensuring the proper sanitisation of ice-cream scoops between use?

Q133 Can my polypropylene cutting boards be put through the dishwasher before routine cleaning?

Q134 How should I store my cutting boards?

Q135 What does the term "clean as you go" mean and how can it best be achieved?

Q136 Is there any benefit from segregation of waste in my business? It seems that the cost of general waste disposal is increasing all the time.

Q137 How can chemical contamination be prevented if chemicals are put onto food surfaces to kill bacteria?

## BARS AND CELLARS

Q138 To what standard should I maintain my cellars structurally, as I understand they are classed as food rooms under the law?

Q139 What are the requirements for bottle stores?

Q140 What facilities with respect to sinks, etc should be provided in my beer store?

Q141 How often should I clean my beer lines?

Q142 What washing facilities do I require in my bar area?

Q143 Why is there a need for a wash-hand basin in a bar area when only low-risk food products are handled?

Q144 Are there any risks from open snacks such as crisps, nuts, pickled onions, gherkins, dips, etc on the bar?

Q145 What is the best method to dispense nuts at the bar to reduce contamination?

Q146 What is the best type of hand-drying facility in bar areas?

Q147 What is the best method of glass storage within the bar area?

Q148 How should I store spirit measures to prevent contamination?

Q149 Is there any risk from selling out-of-date bottled beverages? Am I in breach of any statute if I do so?

Q150 Can I legally recover beers drawn through but not consumed? They appear to be slightly cloudy, particularly at the start and end of the barrel.

Q151 Is there any risk from service of main meals over the bar as well as beverages?

Q152 What may be classed as reasonable protective clothing for use in a bar area?

Q153 What are the rules on smoking in bar areas?

## FOOD HYGIENE TRAINING

Q154 Is there a legal requirement to carry out food hygiene training?

Q155 What recognised training courses are available in food hygiene and who carries them out?

Q156 To what level should I train my staff in food hygiene?

Q157 What subjects should be covered on a basic food safety course undertaken "in-house" within a catering business?

Q158 If food handlers have obtained their basic food hygiene certificate, how frequently should they receive refresher training?

Q159 I have a busy catering organisation and find it extremely difficult to release staff and managers for any training. What are my options?

Q160 How do food hygiene qualifications tie into National Vocational Qualifications (NVQs)?

Q161 What is the best advice to help me pass my Advanced Food Hygiene exams? I have not done an exam for 20 years!

Q162 I am a manager in a catering industry who has only ever done a Basic Food Hygiene course. I have been asked by my boss to do an Advanced Food Hygiene course but confess to being worried about stepping up to that level without doing an Intermediate level first. What are my options?

## FOOD POISONING AND FOOD COMPLAINTS

Q163 Is the increase in reported cases of food poisoning a reflection of greater public awareness or an indication of generally lower standards in catering?

Q164 I have had, on occasions, complaints from customers that they have eaten food which has caused them food poisoning. How can I ascertain whether they are justified and what is the best means by which to deal with such complaints?

Q165 What should I do if I believe food poisoning complaints are justified?

Q166 Is it useful to take food samples of foods that I prepare in case complaints of food poisoning are received?

Q167 What is the benefit of submitting food samples for analysis? What bacteria should I have the food analysed for?

Q168 When should I inform the EHO that my organisation may have caused a food poisoning incident?

Q169 What is the best way of dealing with a customer who finds a foreign object in their food?

Q170 Is it not best to offer a small token in compensation at the table in the case of food complaints?

Q171 What is the true incidence of food poisoning within the UK?

Q172 What is the financial cost of food poisoning in the UK?

## HAZARD ANALYSIS AND ASSURED SAFE CATERING

Q173 I have heard much about HACCP and hazard analysis. What does this mean and is it of any value to my catering business?

Q174 What is the difference between HACCP and hazard analysis?

Q175 What do I need to know about hazard analysis?

Q176 What training should I undertake to carry out my own hazard analysis?

Q177 What should my staff know about hazard analysis?

Q178 How can "critical control points" be easily identified?

Q179 How can my catering business cost-effectively operate a hazard analysis (HACCP) system as required by the regulations?

Q180 What is a practical way of complying with the legal requirements for hazard analysis?

Q181 Is the concept of "assured safe catering" of use to my catering business?

Q182 What will the EHO do if I have not done a hazard analysis for my business?

Q183 What are the key stages in carrying out Hazard Analysis?

Q184 How can hazard analysis in my business be more clearly understood by my staff?

Q185 What, in a few words, is the simplest form of hazard analysis?

Q186 When monitoring a critical point in my catering operation, what should be recorded?

Q187 When should I review my hazard analysis?

Q188 Do I legally have to have a written record of my hazard analysis?

Q189 What are my options if I cannot find the time to carry out hazard analysis myself within my operations?

Q190 When might an EHO seize food and what are my rights in this respect?

Q191 Is it only EHOs who carry out food inspections?

Q192 What records do I need to keep to ensure I have a complete "due diligence" defence?

Q193 What will be the functions of the new Food Standards Agency?

Q194 Where can good, simple guidance on food law be obtained?

## FOOD SAFETY LAW

Q195 In plain language, what laws affect me in the catering business and what do I have to do?

Q196 What are the benefits of the Food Safety Act 1990?

Q197 There have been many changes in food safety legislation. When are we likely to see some stability in this field so that caterers can catch up with those laws which are obviously essential?

Q198 How can I be sure that there will not be further U-turns in Government policy, which have up until now caused much unnecessary expenditure in my catering business?

Q199 Is the concept of all EU countries operating under and within the same hygiene legislation and guidelines an achievable reality or merely a bureaucrat's pipedream which only the UK will sign and enforce?

Q200 Is there a legal requirement to refrigerate eggs?

Q201 I have mice in certain parts of the premises. Will I be closed down by the EHO?

Q202 Is it a legal requirement to use colour-coded chopping boards?

Q203 Are fly-killing machines a legal requirement within premises?

Q204 An environmental health officer recently visited my food business and gave me a Food Safety Act notice requiring work to be carried out. I have insufficient time to do exactly what he requires; what are my options?

Q205 Can I refuse entry to an enforcement officer at times when we are extremely busy and ask them to visit at another time when we are more able to manage and deal with the situation?

Q206 I have received summonses for food hygiene offences which allegedly occurred some time ago with respect to my business. I do not remember when the initial visit was undertaken, but it would appear now that the officer means business. Can they still take a case after such a long time period and what should be my next course of action?

Q207 I understand that Food Safety Act cases are triable both in the magistrates' and crown courts. What would be the better option?

Q208 I run a number of catering businesses in different areas of the country. I have noticed that the requirements of enforcement officers in one area may differ from those of officers in other areas. How can these inconsistencies be eliminated?

Q209 How often do environmental health officers visit food premises and how can I anticipate when I might get an inspection?

Q210 Yesterday my EHO inspected my premises and wasn't very happy to find that some issues which he had written to me about in the past had not been attended to. I tried to tell him that I ordered the parts necessary to comply with his previous letter, but he wouldn't listen. He said he was going to serve a "minded to" notice on me. What does this mean?

Q211 For how long is it recommended that food safety monitoring records be kept?

Q212 How can the catering manager be sure that staff actually follow the guidelines, instructions and policies laid down, apart from requiring them to attend training sessions and to complete and sign the relevant documentation and control forms?

Q213 If I have suspected contamination of food within my catering business, do I have to retain the food and pass it on to the enforcement officer and, if so, how should it be kept prior to return or disposal?

Q214 If high ambient temperatures within kitchens are a food safety risk, why is the law not stricter with respect to controlling ambient temperatures?

Q215 How long can I leave sandwiches out at ambient temperature before I have to dispose of them?

Q216 What major changes did the Food Safety (General Food Hygiene) Regulations 1995 bring about?

Q217 What are the temperature control requirements for caterers under the Food Safety (Temperature Control) Regulations 1995?

Q218 What are the main differences in temperature control regulation in Scotland?

Q219 Do the Food Safety (General Food Hygiene) Regulations 1995 require small businesses to have details of hazard analyses in writing in case the inspector calls?

Q220 The term "adequate" appears open to much debate when considering food hygiene regulations. How can we be sure that we interpret this correctly?

Q221 Surely ISO 9000, the quality standard, would assist environmental health departments throughout the UK to achieve a more uniform inspection standard?

Q222 If butchers' shops now have to be licensed what are the future implications for caterers who do extensive meat preparation?

Q223 What does butchers' shop licensing depend on and is it a guarantee that my butcher is safe?

Q224 What are my legal obligations with respect to labelling menu items that contain peanuts?

Q225 Why is there such a growth in the number of people affected by food allergies?

Q226 How does the concept of "due diligence" under the Food Safety Act 1990 link with hazard analysis?

Q227 I have been asked by my EHO to increase the mobility of my kitchen equipment, to assist cleaning. Can this be insisted upon and are there any options, given the cost of this?

# FOOD SOURCES AND MANUFACTURING

## RED MEAT

**Q1 What potential micro-organisms could be present on meat and what are their origins?**

A All livestock, whether intensively or traditionally reared, carry a whole host of micro-organisms. Many are completely harmless to humans, but others are communicable by coming in contact with animals or by eating their flesh. The following table illustrates the main micro-organism types, sources, mode of spread and method of prevention.

| MICRO-ORGANISMS | TYPE | TYPE OF ANIMAL | MODE OF SPREAD | PREVENTION |
|---|---|---|---|---|
| Salmonella infection | Bacterium | Beef, lamb, pork and deer. | Consumption of infected flesh or milk | Thorough cooking, pasteurisation of milk. |
| Clostridium perfringens | Bacterium | Beef, lamb, pork and deer. | Consumption only — soil bacteria transferred from ground on hooves or hide and onto flesh at abattoir. Minced products provide worst vehicle. | Hygiene at abattoir. Hygiene in the butcher's shop. Care with preparation of diced meat products. |
| Escherichia coli | Bacterium | Beef, lamb, pork, deer and humans. | Consumption of minced meat products, particularly burgers. Close contact with animals, eg on farms. Carried in gut and may be spread in food handling. | Thorough cooking of burgers and other minced products. Good personal hygiene. |

| | | | | |
|---|---|---|---|---|
| Tuberculosis | Bacterium | Cattle, wild animals and humans. | Very rare these days. Mainly infected milk. Person to person and airborne | Statutory testing of herds and use of pasteurised milk. Vaccination, good housing, ventilation and sunlight. |
| Brucellosis (undulant fever, Malta fever) | Brucella abortis | Cattle, sheep and goats. | Very rare, usually confined to farmers and people who consume raw milk and unpasterurised cheese. | Do not drink raw milk or eat unpasteurised cheese. |
| Beef tape worm | Parasite (Taenia saginata) | Cattle | Consumption of uncooked beef and beef products. Steak tartar, rare steak, raw sausage meat. | Do not eat raw beef products. Thorough cooking of beef products. |
| Pork tape worm | Parasite (Taenia solium) | Pigs | Consumption of uncooked pork and pork products. | Do not eat raw pork products. Thorough cooking of pork proudcts. |
| Trichernosis | Parasite (Trichinella spiralis) | Pigs | Pigs kept in unhygienic, rat-infested conditions. | Do not eat raw pork products. Thorough cooking of pork products. |

## Q2 How can I tell if red meat is fit to eat?

A There are a number of indicators which should be studied carefully. These include colour, odour, touch and palpitation.

| INDICATOR | POSSIBLY FIT | POSSIBLY UNFIT |
|---|---|---|
| Colour | Dark red, burgundy red or bright red with white or yellow hard fat. | Green, clear sticky fat. |
| Odour | Fresh aroma, animal-like. | Putrid, decayed, ammonia-like. |
| Touch | Dry or smooth and moist, but not sticky. | Sticky, gritty, shiny. |
| Palpitation | Resilient if depressed. | Depressions stay in place, non-resilient. |
| Other indications | Condition of packaging; clean dry bags or plastic films. | Presence ofrobvious attraction of flies. |

**Q3 How can I tell if frozen red meat is fit to eat?**

A It is very difficult to tell; it would be advisable to defrost the meat to assess its condition.

| INDICATOR | POSSIBLY FIT | POSSIBLY UNFIT |
|---|---|---|
| Colour | Clean, bright appearance, few ice crystals | Ice laden, white frosted, possible appearance of fibrous areas (freezer burn). |
| Shape | Good normal shape for that particular joint. | Distorted for that type of joint — may give the appearance of being re-frozen. |
| Coverings | Good overall covering to protect from frost damage. | Poor, damaged wrappings exposing meat. |

**Q4 How can I tell if vaccum-packed red meat is fit to eat?**

A Whilst vacuum-packed products have a long shelf-life when kept at the required temperature of 0–3°C, without opening vacuum-packed meat it is very difficult to say whether it is fit to eat. When the air is excluded from the meat there is a tendency for the blood to change its form and the meat may be discoloured producing a grey or perhaps green tinge. Only when the air returns and the blood takes this up does the dark or bright red colour return. Temperature abuse will cause anaerobic bacteria (ie bacteria which live without air) to multiply. Some spoilage bacteria may be present and cause the meat to become unfit. Worse still, some anaerobic bacteria may cause serious if not fatal food poisoning, eg botulism. At 0–3°C vacuum-packed meats can be kept for up to two weeks safely and perhaps longer.

## POULTRY

**Q5 Why is raw poultry contaminated with Salmonella?**

A All birds, whether they are chickens, turkeys, geese, ducks or game birds have a high risk of being contaminated by Salmonella organisms. The organism is certainly well established in the food chain and poultry feed was thought to be responsible during the establishment of intensive farming. Up to 80% of poultry could be affected — the caterer should make the assumption that all poultry is contaminated and treat such foods with great care to avoid cross-contamination.

**Q6 Are there any other conditions which may affect poultry that the caterer should be aware of?**

A There are numerous conditions in poultry. However, stringent inspection under the poultry meat regulations should eliminate most if not all of these conditions. The following are some that may still be apparent.

| CONDITION | TYPE OF BIRD | COMMENTS |
|---|---|---|
| "Red Leg" | Chickens. | Has no pathogenic significance to man but has the appearance of uncooked red meat close to the bone even though the poultry has been properly cooked. |
| Breast abscesses | Turkeys and chickens in battery farms. | Caused by cramped cage conditions. Of no real significance and can be trimmed away before cooking. |
| Broken legs and wings | All birds. | Can be seen by infusion of blood or bruising around wings or legs. Such tissue should be cut away. |

**Q7 How can I tell if poultry meat is fit?**

A Poultry meat is reasonably easy to assess because it has had its vital organs, head and feet removed. This causes much disruption to the carcass and potentially much contamination. It will decay rapidly if temperatures are unsatisfactory. The following may be used as a guide to fitness.

| INDICATOR | POSSIBLY FIT | POSSIBLY UNFIT |
|---|---|---|
| Colour | Clean with minimal feathers, white or cream in appearance. | Greening or blotched red is evidence of decay. |
| Shape | Should be plump, well rounded, clean, no distorted or distended areas. | May be emaciated (thin), obvious broken legs or damage. |
| Odour | Clean, fresh smell. | Obvious ammonia-like smell, particularly from cavity. |
| Touch | Resilient if flesh is depressed, with dry surface, not slimy. | Non-resilient and slimy; cavity possibly gritty |
| Coverings | Intact, in-date, good overall protection. | Damaged coverings, excessive drip. |

**Note:** Game birds may give the appearance of being unfit and it is possible that they have been hung for a long period of time. Bacteria have the effect of breaking down tissue producing greening, changes in colour and odour; however, people sometimes like the "gaminess" of such birds. Any presence of mould, larvae or excessive putrefaction should warrant the rejection of game birds, but it is a matter of choice and degree.

## EGGS

**Q8 What is the likelihood of my eggs being contaminated by Salmonella and causing food poisoning?**

A There has been considerable research into Salmonella and eggs. Certainly the recent rise in food poisoning from 1988 onwards has been caused by one particular type of Salmonella, *Salmonella enteritis*, phase type 4. This has now become the most dominant strain of over 2200 different types of Salmonella. It is invasive of poultry and can cross from the bird to the egg leading to low-level contamination, perhaps in the order of 10–20 organisms per egg. This is insufficient to cause food poisoning, but given ambient and prolonged storage conditions of eggs the organisms can multiply to infective levels. Approximately 1% of egg-laying birds contain Salmonella, with less than 3% of eggs affected by individual infected hens.

When food is batch processed, eg during the production of food products like mayonnaise, mousse, hollandaise sauce, etc, large number of eggs are used and the likelihood of infection of the whole batch is increased. When such foods are then stored at incorrect ambient temperatures the chances of food poisoning are heightened; many classic cases of food poisoning have occurred as a result of these circumstances.

**ACTION PLAN TO PREVENT SALMONELLA FOOD POISONING FROM EGGS**

- Purchase eggs from known, reputable suppliers.
- Store egs under temperature control within the kitchen.
- Properly stock rotate eggs. Use within one week of purchase.
- Do not prepare foods in which the egg is not going to be cooked, eg mayonnaise, mousse, etc.
- Use pasteurised eggs where raw egg is required.

**Q9 Are free-range eggs better than battery-farm eggs?**

A There is no evidence to support this. Eggs contain a high level of protein at the same levels either way. Battery-farmed eggs are likely to be cleaner and better in terms of quality control. Smallholding farm eggs may be dirty, old (ie may not have been noticed first time around), cracked or otherwise soiled, which may give rise to contamination within the kitchen. In terms of Salmonella infection, there is no evidence to support the fact that they are less contaminated — the Salmonella organism is ubiquitous.

**Q10 What are the alternatives to using fresh-shell eggs?**

A Because of the spate of food poisoning outbreaks associated with eggs, food manufacturers introduced processing methods which can guarantee freedom from Salmonella and other organisms. Pasteurised eggs can be a useful alternative. They are heat-treated to around 64°C which does not solidify the egg but destroys pathogenic organisms including Salmonella. Dried egg is also a most useful product. Having had the water removed and pathogenic organisms destroyed it has a long shelf-life providing it is kept dry. Frozen liquid egg is also a valuable food ingredient which has a long shelf-life under frozen conditions. It has also been pasteurised to destroy micro-organisms. Both yolk and albumin can be supplied separately or in combination. It should be remembered though that any fresh product which has been pasteurised may still contain non-pathogenic spoilage organisms which reduces its shelf-life. Care should be taken to ensure good stock rotation and avoid risk of contamination.

## MILK AND CREAM

**Q11 Is it safe to drink raw milk and cream?**

A There are certain consumers and certain farmers who promote the consumption of raw (unpasteurised) milk and cream. Whilst there have been many improvements in animal husbandry and farming practice in terms of hygiene, raw milk and cream remain a serious potential public health risk which cannot be underestimated. Much depends on the regular testing of herds for such diseases as Tuberculosis and Brucellosis; however, animals can contract a number of infections including

Salmonella, Campylobacter and Clostridium perfringens. There are also a large amount of potential contaminants to milk from the environment in which the animals are kept and from the herdsmen and dairymen who control the animals. The following is a list of potential infections in milk and cream.

| INFECTION | ORGANISM | SOURCE OF CONTAMINATION | OCCURRENCE | METHOD OF CONTROL |
|---|---|---|---|---|
| Tuberculosis | | Direct from animals which may be infected by other wild animals. | Not common. More common overseas. | Regular testing of herds. Pasteurisation of milk. |
| Brucellosis | Brucella abortis | Stock animals and wild animals. | Rare in the UK — more common overseas particularly in Mediterranean and tropical countries. | Vaccination of cattle, regular milk sampling and pasteurisation. |
| Salmonella | Salmonella | Animal feed, birds and wild fowl, humans. | Common but not often milk-borne. | Care with disposal of human waste. Salmonella-free animal feeds. Control of environment with respect to fowl. Exclusion of infected food handlers from dairy work. |
| Campylo-bacter | Campylo-bacterenteritis and Campylobacter jejuni | Animals and environment. Birds,wild fowl. | Common. Some milk-borne outbreaks still occur. | Good animal husbandry. Control of wild fowl around cattle. Prevention of contamination of milk; pasteurisation. |
| Clostridium perfringens | Clostridium perfringens | Environment — particularly hide, hooves, faecal matter. | Common. | Good hygienic design of farms, lerages, etc. Regular cleaning and hygiene of animals. Care in the dairy to avoid contamination risks. |

| | | | | |
|---|---|---|---|---|
| Listeriosis | Listeria monocytogenes | Environmental. | Common in foods made of milk. | Dairy hygiene, cleaning of animals, etc. Milk pasteurisation. |

The above list is by no means exhaustive and there are many more infections, including Staphylococcus aureus from food handlers that may cause difficulties. It is not advisable to drink raw milk or use it within catering premises. In Scotland it has been banned by regulations, but in Britain raw milk can be obtained direct from farms and is normally for private use. It may be encountered when camping or in country areas at events, etc. Caterers are strongly advised not to use it.

**Q12 How is milk heat-treated?**

A Milk is heat-treated by a number of methods which include the following.

| METHOD | TEMPERATURE AND TIME | NUTRITIONAL VALUE | ORGANISMS DESTROYED | ORGANISMS REMAINING |
|---|---|---|---|---|
| Pasteurisation | High temperature and short time (HTST). 72.5°C for 15 seconds. | Same | All pathogenic organisms including Salmonella, Brucellosis, Tuberculosis, Campylo-bacter, etc. | Most spoilage organisms that are "thermophal" (heat-loving) including Lactobacilli, Bacillus stearothermophilus. |
| Sterilisation | Boiling 10-30 minutes | Affected | None remaining until container is opened. | |
| Ultra heat treatment | 130°C for 1 second | Affected | All | None |

The higher the temperatures, the more organisms are destroyed and nutritional value affected.

**Q13 Why does pasteurised milk still have a limited shelf-life even within a refrigerator?**

A Pasteurised milk contains many spoilage organisms, which turn the milk sour and assist in its curdling or clumping hence its visual appearance after a few days in the refrigerator. The colder the temperature it is kept at, and the less variation it receives during delivery and whilst being prepared, the longer the shelf-life. It should be recognised, however, that once a container is opened bacteria from the packaging and the environment will contaminate milk and quickly make it go off.

## CHEESE

**Q14 With so many cheeses available how can I assess the fitness and safety of cheese?**

A Many cheeses are "alive" and have been ripened by mould and bacteria. These are essentially spoilage organisms which have been introduced to provide characteristic flavour and ageing. Whilst it is normal for blue cheese to be veined with blue mould it would not be normal to see similar blue mould on cheddar. Other indications of unfitness may be the ballooning of packaging, the sliminess created by certain types of bacteria and tastes of rancidity from oxidation of fats. Bacterial contamination is not visible and certainly the buyer must beware. Any unpasteurised cheeses may contain organisms including Salmonella, Campylobacter, Listeria and perhaps Brucellosis. Cheeses from the Mediterranean islands have been known to be contaminated in the past. Unpasteurised cheese should be avoided in mass catering situations. Cheese should be kept refrigerated once it has been cut as this is a point at which contamination can be introduced.

**Q15 I have heard much about soft cheeses being contaminated by Listeria organisms. How does this occur and how can the infection be prevented?**

A Soft cheeses are ripened by either bacteria or moulds and they are often left in damp cellars for many months if not years. The dust in the environment collects on the surfaces of such cheeses and when they are further processed or prepared or cut from the whole, the cheese becomes contaminated from its outer surface. Listeria is an organism which can be described as a food-borne infection. This means only a small number of organisms may cause an illness. Multiplication of Listeria bacterium can be extremely slow. The following advice should be followed.

- Storage of soft cheeses at below 5°C is recommended; however, the organisms can multiply at temperatures below 3°C.
- Once cheeses are cut they should be properly refrigerated.
- Pregnant women should not eat soft cheeses (they have shown to be predisposed to the illness caused by Listeria).
- Only small amounts of soft cheese should be brought out for service.
- It is normal to serve soft cheese at ambient temperatures; providing it is freshly prepared and in limited quantity it is safe to do so.

Good stock rotation of soft cheeses is essential.

## VEGETABLES

**Q16 How can I ensure the quality and freshness of fruit and vegetables for my catering operation?**

A There are a number of considerations which should help.

- Choose a good supplier who will deliver daily. Inspect the supplier's premises and assess the handling procedures, ensuring that care in handling is undertaken.
- Do not over-order — careful planning and liaison with the supplier is necessary.
- Check produce on arrival for freshness and quality — do not accept anything that is not of the expected standard.
- Ensure that menus are planned with use of seasonal vegetables and fruit.
- Take care with handling of delivered vegetables and ensure that they are stored in a well-ventilated cold store, off the floor and with good air circulation.
- Remove any fruit and vegetables from their plastic films and packaging — such storage is not good for the longevity of the produce.
- Ensure any damaged or perished items are removed the moment they are discovered, as such items may result in spoilage of other undamaged produce.

**Q17 What causes fruit and vegetables to spoil?**

A There are a number of factors to consider, but certainly age and damage allow the following to gain a hold and destroy these foods.

| FACTOR | EFFECT |
|---|---|
| Spoilage bacteria, yeast, mould | Yeast and mould are evident by the dark sunken patches and green/blue growth on the outside surface. |
| | Yeast can produce carbon monoxide gas and alcoholic flavours. |
| | Initial effects are limpness and shrinkage. Taste is affected and vitamin content reduced. |
| Enzymes | These are naturally occurring chemicals which can be produced by bacteria and upon the death of cells. They produce soft rot, perhaps brown in colour. |
| Pests | Insects, including fruit flies, can detect rotting fruit and vegetables from a distance. They may bring along other spoilage micro-organisms and lay eggs which will hatch, producing larvae which will consume the foods. |

**Q18 Are organic foods more safe than the mass-produced foods?**

A This is difficult to answer: there are many issues at work here and many learned people who claim pesticides, hormones and antibiotic residues will eventually prove harmful in the long term by producing health effects in humans. There is a need for considerable research to support this theory. Nevertheless it is common sense to avoid such substances wherever possible. Organic food is not likely to be more nutritious and will have blemishes and a poorer appearance and there will be a need for more washing and preparation. There may be a heightened risk of soil bacteria such as Listeria and E.coli but proper composting methods on farms should reduce this risk. Perhaps the best answer is that there is no gain without a little pain and organic foods will have the edge over chemically produced crops in the long run.

**Q19 There has been much in the news about E.coli 0157. Is this a new organism and where does it come from?**

A It is believed that it is a relatively new strain of the well-established E.coli bacterium and has probably been around for the last 20 years or so. It is causing around 1000 cases per year in the UK and has quickly established itself around the world. The main source is the intestines of our food animals, particularly sheep and cattle, and they contaminate the farms where they are reared. It can be contracted directly from contact with faecal matter and children have been known to develop it from farm visits. There are also cases reported from pop festivals where the ground has been churned by pedestrian traffic, and also from beaches. The main foods from which it has spread are milk, cooked meats (by cross-contamination) in restaurants, caterers and butchers, cheese, fruit juice, burgers and a whole host of other foods often not thoroughly cooked.

**Q20 What are the implications of the dioxin contamination of food during the 1999 Belgian food incident?**

A It is believed that dioxins are chemicals which may cause cancer and levels were found in meat and milk products above those judged acceptable for human consumption. It is not believed that anyone was made ill from this incident and the source of the contamination is understood to be animal food contaminated by engine oil. All the Belgian foods affected at the time were withdrawn by a food hazard warning. However, the Belgian government was slow in letting everyone know about the laboratory tests and findings and as a result resigned from power. It is likely that much of the contaminated food has been consumed.

# VEGETARIAN FOODS

**Q21 What are the main bacterial risks with vegetarian catering, considering that meat, poultry and fish are not used?**

A Due consideration must be given to the other ingredients in vegetarian meals, especially eggs, milk and cheese, which are widely used in vegetarian cooking. While the selective nature of vegetarianism does preclude rather a large number of particular bacteria, food sources are not the only origin. Environmental pests and human origins still have a part to play and the main bacterial contaminants which may occur are shown in the table below.

| BACTERIA | TYPES OF FOODS | PREVENTION |
|---|---|---|
| Salmonella | Eggs, unpasteurised cheese, untreated milk, chocolate and possibly soft fruits including raspberries and melon. | Use of pasteurised liquid or frozen egg, pasteurised cheeses, care with food handling. |
| Bacillus cereus | Rice,wheat and other cereals. | Thorough washing prior to cooking, temperature control of prepared food products. |
| Clostridium perfringens | Usually a soil contaminant, therefore vegetables are often highly contaminated. | Thorough washing of salads and other vegetables before preparation. |
| Campylobacter | Raw milk | Only use treated milk. May also be in pasteurised milk, contamination from birds and animals. Care needed with receipt of deliveries. |
| Escherichia coli | All salad foods may be contaminated | Thorough washing — levels of contamination in low-risk vegetable foods would not usually cause illness. |
| Listeria monocytogenes | Prepared salads | Thorough washing — levels of contamination in low-risk vegetable foods would not usually cause illness. |

| | | |
|---|---|---|
| Shigella sonnei (dysentery) | Prepared salads, water and milk. | Thorough washing — levels of contamination in low-risk vegetable foods would not usually cause illness. Personal hygiene very important. |

**Q22 Why is it necessary to pre-soak dry pulses prior to cooking?**

A A common mistake made by those preparing kidney beans, and other such foods, is to cook them without thorough soaking to remove toxins which are often found to be naturally occurring. Pre-soaking for 24 hours removes these toxins. The water must be discarded before the cooking process. The toxin causes a short-duration gastroenteritis.

# FOOD PRESERVATION

**Q23 Are there any risks from the use and consumption of irradiated foods?**

A No. Research has shown that there are no risks at normal irradiation doses and recent changes in the law have made irradiation of food possible in the UK. It is accepted in many countries throughout the world. There is no alteration to nutritional value or the nature of the food.

**Q24 Should I always purchase foods which do not contain additives?**

A Only a small number of additives are unnecessary within food in that they impart bright colours or perhaps improve palatability and texture. Most additives perform a most valuable role in preventing spoilage and food poisoning. Many are quite "natural" and without additives there certainly would be more food poisoning and complaints about food.

**Q25 What can the caterer do to extend the life of food?**

A There are a number of methods which can be employed from simple refrigeration or freezing to methods such as bottling, vacuum-packing or the use of preservatives. It should be a principle that foods be used as quickly as possible and continuity of supply ensured. Some methods, particularly vacuum-packing, may be hazardous if guaranteed hygienic conditions are not observed.

**Q26 Why is vacuum-packing hazardous?**

A Ideal conditions are created by the process of vacuum-packing for the multiplication of the bacterium Clostridium botulinum, which produces one of the deadliest toxins known to man — botulism. If dirt, dust or filth is incorporated into vacuum-packed food and conditions of ambient storage occur, then botulism is possible. There are, however, few documented cases of this. Generally, only raw foods should be vacuum-packed and they should be kept refrigerated.

**Q27 Why should I use preserved foods when so much fresh food is available?**

A There are a number of points in favour of preserved foods which include the following.

- Out-of-season foods such as asparagus, strawberries, etc can be made available all year round.
- Continuity of supplies is established, perhaps for infrequent deliveries.
- There are bulk purchase and cost implications to be considered.
- There is less likelihood of serious health risk, eg pasteurised eggs.
- Certain dishes lend themselves better to preserved foods, eg fruit cakes.
- Consistency is ensured with equal portion sizes.

**Q28 What is meant by "ambient temperature" and how can convenience foods be preserved so they can be stored at such temperatures?**

A "Ambient" means room temperature and depends on the climatic conditions prevailing at any time. In the summer, room temperature may be between 16–25°C and in the winter perhaps between 5–16°C depending on the location in the building. There are many foods which can be stored at ambient temperatures. Generally they are all preserved by factory processing and include canned goods, dried foods, bottled goods, and foods which have been sterilised including sterilised milk and cream in hermetically sealed containers.

Other examples might include foods which have been pickled, brined or where sugar has been added in the case of jams and sauces, including cranberry sauce. Many fruits can be transformed into candy foods also by adding sugar; these often make good breakfast cereal additives. Chocolate may also be stored at ambient temperature as it is completely dry in nature. There are many sauces that are preserved by virtue of adding vinegar but it is a general rule that when any sauce or jar is opened it should then be refrigerated, as deterioration may occur once air has got to the product. Temperature control is always good practice, particularly with high-protein foods, including mayonnaise and other sauces.

To store foods at ambient temperature there are a number of general principles which should be followed. These include:

- complete removal of moisture by drying in the oven or sun-drying (this is not usually undertaken in the UK but may be used for fish in the tropics)
- bottling in vinegar — this is useful for pickled eggs, boiled eggs and vegetables
- production of preserves by adding vast quantities of sugar to boiled fruits
- lowering of the pH by addition of citric or acetic acid (vinegar or lime juice).

One would have to be very sure of the quantities and type of food if storage at ambient temperature was the ultimate objective.

# GENETICALLY MODIFIED FOODS

**Q29 What are genetically modified foods and can they be harmful to health?**

A Cells contain genetic information which determine their characteristics and those of any progeny. This information is held in genes which are made up of DNA. By changing the structure of the genes it is possible to stop unwanted characteristics. For instance, tomatoes can be genetically modified to last longer. There has been a case in the past where soya beans were modified with Brazil nut protein which was a potential problem for those with nut allergies. The jury is still out on this one.

**Q30 How can I best ensure I am not being supplied with food that has genetically modified ingredients?**

A You should send your suppliers a questionnaire or ask them to certify that their products do not contain genetically modified (GM) ingredients. There is also a growing band of food manufacturers who are declaring that their food products are GM free.

If you have concerns it may be wise to use one of these manufacturers as an alternative. A simple test kit is currently being developed in order to detect GM products but is not yet available.

**Q31 What training should be given to my staff about genetically modified foods?**

A Essentially they need to know what products may contain GM ingredients so that they can advise your customers if asked. This is an alternative option to labelling which , if done, would negate the need for training.

**Q32 What genetically modified foods are approved for human consumption?**

A Tomatoes, soya and maize are at the moment approved for human consumption. They are often used as ingredients within manufactured foods. It has been a legal requirement since 1 September 1998 to label products that contain GM foods.

**Q33 What are my legal obligations with respect to labelling of menu items containing genetically modified foods?**

A From 18 September 1999 there was a legal requirement under the Food Labelling (Amendment) Regulations 1999 to ensure customers are provided with advice as to which foods for sale may contain GM material. This can be done with notices saying "Products on the menu marked with an asterisk contain ingredients produced from genetically modified soya" or "The following foods sold in this establishment contain ingredients produced from genetically modified soya and/or maize". Alternatively, you may, in the case of non-permanent menus, e.g. chalk boards, write "Some products in the establishment contain ingredients produced from genetically modified soya/maize. Please ask the staff for further details." In this case you will need to ensure your staff are trained and updated as to your situation on GM foods.

**Q34 How are GM foods approved for safety?**

A In the UK there is an advisory group known as the Advisory Committee on Novel Foods and Processes (ACNFP). They are independent experts with a worldwide knowledge of this field. They assess by the process known as "substantial equivalence" which involves a comparison of a GM food with its conventional equivalent and a detailed examination of any differences. This approach has been endorsed by the World Health Organization and is widely used around the world. Any novel food not used in the UK before has to go before the committee and extensive research is undertaken.

# FOOD SUPPLY

**Q35 What should I check if I carry out a "due diligence" audit of one of my suppliers?**

A All audits should be biased toward food safety management. In order to carry out a worthwhile audit it would be important to draw up an inspection format prior to the visit along the following lines.

| ITEMS INSPECTED | SATIS. | UNSATIS. | ACTION TAKEN |
|---|---|---|---|
| **Food Safety Management**<br>Due diligence records and procedures | | | |
| Hazard analysis/Food safety policy | | | |
| Staff training/Records | | | |
| Product recall arrangements | | | |
| **Premises**<br>General cleanliness of food rooms | | | |
| Maintenance standards of walls, floor, ceiling surfaces | | | |
| Condition of location of sinks, wash-hand basins, soap, towel, lighting, ventilation, toilet facilities | | | |
| **Food Handling**<br>Use of sanitisers | | | |
| Temperature control | | | |
| Evidence of cross contamination | | | |
| Use of refrigerators | | | |
| Cleanliness | | | |
| Availability of wash-hand facilities (soap, towel, nailbrush) | | | |
| First-aid facilities | | | |
| Condition of working clothing | | | |
| Provision of lockers for outdoor clothing | | | |
| Report of infections procedure | | | |
| General appearance of staff | | | |

| | | | |
|---|---|---|---|
| **Waste Disposal and Handling**<br>Lidded bins | | | |
| External areas | | | |
| **Pest Control**<br>Evidence of pests | | | |
| Fly screening | | | |

**Q36 I do not feel experienced enough to do my company's supplier audits. What are my options?**

A One way to deal with this is to employ a specialist consultant in food safety to carry out the checks for you. These consultants are usually qualified EHOs in the private sector. They will be able to supply you with the technical expertise required to carry out such an audit and will provide a detailed report on the standards of the supplier (including any recommendations). However, if you do not wish to take this approach, you can train a member of staff to carry out such audits — Advanced Food Hygiene would be the minimum requirement for this.

**Q37 What should I check when receiving deliveries?**

A There are a number of matters which are important.

- Whether products are within the date code specified.
- Whether products are within the temperature parameters of –18°C for frozen goods and below 4°C for chilled goods. It may be possible to accept deliveries at slightly higher temperatures, say –15°C for frozen goods and 8°C for chilled goods if this only occurs on a one-off basis. If temperatures are regularly outside of the safe parameters, you must bring it to the attention of your supplier and request that all future deliveries meet your specifications.
- Any signs of damage or dampness to containers.
- Any signs of pest infestation.
- Quality of the produce.
- Products are of the correct weight, quantity and type required.

All this should be checked against the purchase order. Products should be accepted *only* if satisfactory.

**Q38 How often should I have food delivered for my catering operation?**

A This depends entirely on the type of produce required, the quality of the food to be served and also the nature of the supplier. It may also depend on your location within the country. Some areas can only be supplied once or twice a week, whilst others in major conurbations would find it easier to obtain food supplies. In general terms, the following is usually necessary:

- vegetables and fruit daily or each second day
- fish daily or each second day
- meat daily or each second day
- frozen foods twice a week or weekly
- dry foods once a week.

It should be remembered that stored food perishes and also costs money. Efforts should be made to keep food stocks to a minimum. Seven days' supplies for most non-perishable foods is usually satisfactory.

**Q39 What shall I do if one of my suppliers is prosecuted for hygiene offences?**

A This is certainly a bad sign. It demonstrates that the hygiene or food safety of that supplier is in question. Depending on the circumstances it may be best to make a visit to the premises and to gain assurances that matters have been attended to and future supplies will be of a good standard. In extreme cases it may be necessary to delist the supplier and go elsewhere.

**Q40 What should I do if I receive a complaint from a customer that I believe to be a supplier problem?**

A You have two options:

- go to the environmental health officer and explain the situation, or
- go to the supplier and investigate the occurrence thoroughly.

A letter to the customer stating that the issue complained of is a supplier problem which has been corrected may be enough to satisfy that customer. However, you may still have to demonstrate that you took all "reasonable precautions" and showed "due diligence" if not.

**Q41 The concept of due diligence appears to require my organisation to audit our suppliers and it occurs to me that all other organisations are doing a similar task. Why can we not pool our meagre resources and have all suppliers audited and approved centrally rather than carrying out so many visits individually?**

A What a good question! Large-volume food suppliers must by now be receiving literally hundreds of visits from their clients and having to cope with the deluge of requests and herds of inspectors wandering around the plants offering varying standards of advice and requirements. It also seems rather odd that small companies should send in their chefs or food and beverage managers to audit large companies which have far better and more professional resources in-house. One rule of thumb may be that only audits of companies smaller than the investigating company should be undertaken by clients.

There is no reason why companies cannot band together and have their common suppliers audited. This would save much time and effort for all parties and allow caterers to get on with managing their businesses. There is scope for some form of national supplier agency with guarantees of quality. This concept is known as "third party accreditation" and is currently under development. Certainly if a company employed qualified consultants to carry out regular audits of suppliers then this will help to reassure caterers of the quality of food that they provide.

**Q42 Is the purchase of pre-prepared and pre-packed raw meats and vegetables a safer and more hygienic option than on-site preparation in the kitchen and, if so, is the increased cost a fair reflection of the contamination/food poisoning risks avoided?**

A This depends on the quality of food expected and the type of operation undertaken. It is likely, for example, that high-class restaurants would wish to be more involved with the detailed preparation of each item of food, whereas commercial catering operations (which often work to a tight price per head) may not be so reluctant to be involved with issues such as mass production and mass volumes. Commercial caterers would perhaps be more concerned about the possible loss of a contract in the event of a food poisoning case, which might affect not only the particular unit where the catering is being undertaken but also other client operations.

Certainly many of the cross-contamination risks presented by preparing meat and vegetables can be eliminated by the use of pre-prepared and pre-packed foods and therefore food poisoning potential is reduced. There are few catering operations anywhere which butcher large carcasses of meat in any event and certainly ready-prepared vegetables are gaining a hold in many catering operations.

In terms of cost-effectiveness the following must be taken into account:

- staff costs for preparing the food, eg cutting, washing, slicing, etc
- premises costs, eg in terms of food preparation space saved which does not have to be cleaned and costs of machinery that is no longer required, eg potato peelers, mixers, bandsaws, etc
- a change in the size of refrigerated storage needed; sliced vegetables will have to be stored under refrigeration as well as meat products
- reduced waste and risk of drains blocking, wear and tear on waste disposal units, reduction in volume of waste for collection, etc.

It is the dirty processes which certainly bring the greatest risks into catering operations and anything that will reduce these risks has to be beneficial.

# FOOD STORAGE

**Q43 How can I get the best from my food storage facilities?**

A The aim should be to store the minimum food necessary. Keep food at its maximum freshness, ensuring good stock rotation and generally assist the quality of the finished product. This can be achieved by the following measures.

- Good storage environment — freezers and refrigerators should operate at the correct temperatures, ie –18°C and 1 to 4°C respectively. Dry stores should be cool, dry and well ventilated.
- All products should be covered to prevent contamination. Any partly used products should be labelled with date opened and contents. All products should be stored off the floor irrespective of their location. Products should be easy to find and easy to stock rotate.
- No refrigerator or freezer should be overloaded. Chest freezers can be a menace in this respect. There is need for good air circulation around products.
- There should be no risks of cross-contamination, particularly within the refrigerator.
- All refrigerators and freezers require regular defrosting and cleaning.
- Twice a year (autumn and spring) professional servicing to ensure cold storage works effectively throughout the year and minimises the chance of a breakdown.

**Q44 What is "freezer burn"?**

A This is a condition of frozen food which occurs when it is not properly wrapped and covered. It occurs when either frozen food is exposed or it is slowly frozen from fresh. Large ice crystals form which break up the texture of the food. The ice often evaporates from the product exposing dull, fibrous patches of the food. The food can change its texture and colour considerably — meat and beefburgers can be a grey, fibrous colour instead of a natural pink or red colour. The quality of such food will be considerably reduced and may be unfit for human consumption.

**Q45 Why can refrigerated foods be stored quite legally at 8°C when clearly this is in the danger zone?**

A Good question. Pathogenic and spoilage bacteria can grow slowly at below 8°C. However, the legislation that sets this level is as a result of EU law, which has attempted to unify standards. The 8°C standard is seen as being an achievable target for all Member States while still providing a reasonable level of safety. In the UK, guidance recommends that a temperature of 5°C is achieved and your hazard analysis should take account of this.

**Q46 I notice small flies in my vegetable storage area. What are they and how can I get rid of them?**

A These are likely to be Drosophila (fruit flies). They occur in such areas when perished and rotten food is available to them. The cleaning standards may not be what they should be and also there may be perished food under shelving or within unnoticed bags. The following will reduce the incidence of these flies:

- daily checking of all food stocks and removal of perished products
- regular cleaning and removal of products which have fallen on the floor
- cool and ventilated conditions
- high standard of maintenance and cleaning.

**Q47 What foods need to be stored under refrigeration?**

A The **Food Safety (Temperature Control) Regulations 1995** require that "food which is likely to support the growth of pathogenic organisms or the formation of toxins" is kept under refrigeration. These high-risk foods tend to be high in protein and are ready to be eaten. Examples include cooked meats, cooked vegetables, soft cheeses, smoked or cured fish and any cooked dish containing egg or cheese. Many raw foods (such as meat) are not classified as high risk, as the cooking process should kill off any harmful bacteria.

**Q48 What are the rules on storing boxes within freezers and refrigerators?**

A Boxes within freezers are generally not a hazard and can safely be placed on shelving, particularly within large walk-in freezers. In refrigerators, boxes tend to become moist and can come into contact with other prepared foods; when one considers they have been transported on the back of a vehicle and perhaps been on the floor there may be a considerable risk. All foods should be unpacked from such wrappings and the wrappings should be discarded at an early stage.

**Q49 I have heard the term "double stacking" mentioned with respect to refrigerators. What does it mean and how can I prevent it?**

A Double stacking is when food containers are placed on top of each other, directly on top of the food, generally because of limited space within refrigerators. Contamination from the bottom of the container can get onto the top of the food which only has one last line of defence, ie cooking, to reduce that contamination. Foreign matter, eg glass, splinters, metal, etc could be passed from the container to the food and obviously would remain on the food through to service if not noticed. The problem can be prevented in the following ways.

- More shelving being purchased within refrigerators provided there is sufficient room for more. Often they are supplied only with five shelves. There is no reason why 10 or even 15 shelves cannot be obtained under these circumstances.
- Ensuring that all containers are lidded.
- Placing greaseproof paper over the food before double stacking. (However, this should be considered only as a last resort.)

**Q50 What should I do if a freezer breaks down?**

A This depends on when the breakdown was noticed. A temperature check should be undertaken of the frozen produce. If the breakdown has just occurred and the food has not been affected, then it may be possible to transfer the frozen goods under close supervision to another freezer; these circumstances are perfectly safe. If products have defrosted then there is the option of cooking the food provided that the temperature rise has not been above 5°C and provided that the food is used that day. If the food has risen to an inordinate temperature, above 5°C, then it may be better to discard the food and make a claim on insurance if this is available. For this to be undertaken it will be necessary to get an independent note of the loss. Local council environmental health officers may perform this service for a fee; however, independent consultants are also available.

**Q51 How often should I defrost my chest freezers?**

A At least every month would be preferable. However, it depends on how often the unit is opened and products removed or restocked.

**Q52 How often should I check the temperature of my refrigerators?**

A There is no legal requirement to carry out this action, with the exception of transport and temporary premises. However, it is certainly good practice in terms of due diligence. Some organisations would suggest three times a day but this could be considered by some to be rather an onerous requirement; twice a day will normally suffice. The food temperature should be monitored and not the air temperature. This should be undertaken with a digital-type metal probe thermometer. Infra-red non-contact thermometers are now available which give a quick and reliable warning. There are automatic devices, namely the "plastic chicken", which can be placed within the unit and remotely monitored, but such devices are expensive.

There is little point in monitoring the dial readouts on refrigerators and freezers as these are notoriously unreliable and generally only measure air temperature.

**Q53 How long will food last under refrigeration and within freezers?**

A This entirely depends on temperature. The colder the temperature, the longer food will last. At –18°C quality will be preserved for at least six months and perhaps one year. At 1°C there will be no adverse changes for around five days. A recommended shelf-life within refrigerators should be a maximum of two to three days.

**Q54 Is there any value in labelling refrigerators and shelving to ensure risks of cross-contamination are prevented?**

A Certainly if there is sufficient space it is a most worthwhile exercise. Wherever possible, raw and cooked products should be kept in separate refrigerators and if space is limited raw products should be kept below cooked foods. All foods should be kept covered. Labelling shelving may prove useful; however, the material used for labelling should be such that it is easily washable and not easily detached.

**Q55 With all the publicity regarding E.coli 0157 in meat, do I now have to keep raw meat separate from cooked products?**

A Yes. The **Food Safety (General Food Hygiene) Regulations 1995** require that "food is protected against any contamination likely to render the food injurious to health." Environmental Health Officers are now required to inspect more frequently those premises that put food at risk from contamination with E.coli 0157. If possible, raw meat should be stored in a separate refrigerator from high-risk ready-to-eat foods. Failing this, the old rule of storing raw foods below the cooked applies. The law does not require separate storage areas, although this may be introduced in the future.

**Q56 I have limited space within my dry store. Why do I have to keep food off the floor?**

A Although this is not a legal requirement there are a number of main reasons why food should be stored off the floor.

- While the floor is being cleaned (particularly by mopping), boxes containing food may become damp — this dampness will penetrate through the boxes and affect the food.
- Condensation and dampness may be a problem in any case even if precautions are taken to protect the boxes during cleaning.
- Dirt from the floor adheres to the base of boxes and is often transferred onto kitchen worktops.
- Pest harbourage is created at the back of boxes and a dirt trap is formed which is difficult to access.

**Q57 I have only a limited dry store facility which is a long way from the kitchen. Why can I not use the kitchen for day-to-day dry storage?**

A Many kitchens suffer because of poor dry storage facilities. They become cluttered with every shelf and area under food preparation surfaces covered with dry products. These get dusty and greasy and the products become damp from the humid environment of the kitchen. No food products should be stored within kitchens. It is not a storage area and only the food being prepared should be present. Even sauces, wines, etc should be removed on trays to the dry store once the day's production has been completed. Storing food within the kitchens can prevent effective cleaning and lead to pest harbourage.

**Q58 Where should I store eggs?**

A There are a number of schools of thought with respect to eggs. A certain number of eggs will contain Salmonella organisms at low levels and therefore, in order to prevent multiplication of these organisms in what is a high-protein situation, all eggs should be stored under refrigeration. Deliveries should be made frequently to a catering premises and there should be an effort to turn over stock extremely quickly. Eggs can be brought up to ambient temperature for preparation as this may be necessary in certain situations such as baking. Whenever possible a change from shell eggs to pasteurised eggs should be made in the interest of safety.

**Q59 What temperature should ice cream be kept at if I wish to scoop it straight from the tub?**

A Frozen food temperature is generally –18°C. However, for short-term storage ice cream can be stored in a "conservator" at –12°C. Remember to put the lids back on to prevent melting.

**Q60 How can I tell the freshness of shellfish supplies?**

A All shellfish should be clean, as free as possible from "beard". They should be closed shut and have a fresh smell and appearance. Any damaged shellfish should be discarded.

**Q61 How can I tell the freshness of crabs and lobsters?**

A They should be alive. Be careful of the pincers!

**Q62 How should I store fresh fish?**

A Fresh fish is a notoriously sensitive product. When one considers the filleting process large numbers of bacteria will have been exposed to the fish flesh and putrefaction occurs extremely quickly if the temperature is permitted to become too high. All fish should therefore be stored in melting ice at 0–1°C and a special refrigerator should be purchased for the purpose. Under no circumstances should fish be stored above 2 or 3°C, as the product may quickly become unfit for human consumption.

**Q63 What is the best method of storing poultry to prevent risk of contamination?**

A Poultry is a highly contaminated product which should always be stored on the bottom shelf, even below red meat, as a priority. All turkeys, chickens, ducks, etc should be stored on trays covered and away from other foods.

**Q64 If I purchase a bought-in wrapped meat pie with a "use by" date on the product and I do not use it or sell it, can I freeze it for sale on another occasion, providing I do so before the "use by" date?**

A There may be little food safety risk from undertaking this activity, if any. The issues are those of compliance with food labelling requirements and also food quality. Home freezing is a practice which should be discouraged in any event, particularly of food approaching the end of its safe useful life. Domestic freezers are not capable of freezing quickly, therefore damage is caused to the food by the formation of large ice crystals (see Q44 on "freezer burn"). Obviously if food has a "use by" date and the product is frozen there is no doubt that the product will be used later than the date stated. Enforcement officers and the general public are likely to require an explanation of why such a bad practice was adopted. Only food which is purchased frozen should be kept frozen and all foods bought with a "use by" date should be sold within that date in order to remain within present food safety laws.

**Q65 What is the difference between yoghurts which can be stored at room temperature and those which have to be refrigerated?**

A Certain desserts can be stored outside of temperature control if they have a pH (ie the measure of acidity or alkalinity) below 4.5. Products with such a pH are quite acid and this creates an environment where bacteria find it difficult to grow. Coupled with the fact that such products may be made from sterilised milk and prepared under extremely hygienic conditions, the bacterial load is likely to be extremely low and therefore the product would have a shelf-life outside of refrigeration.

# PERSONAL HYGIENE

**Q66 How long does a person remain infectious after having suffered from food poisoning?**

A This depends entirely on the type of infection that has been suffered. Salmonella is of particular concern; in these circumstances people can carry the organisms for many months, if not years. With other infections sufferers may be clear in a matter of days. There is a legal requirement for any person suffering from Salmonella to submit three clear faecal specimens consecutively before they can be considered clear and fit for food handling. Sufferers of viral gastroenteritis are highly infectious while they have the symptoms but after three to seven days their infectivity reduces considerably. Such persons should refrain from work for at least three days before recommencing food handling and should not do so at all without the consent of their general practitioner. For Campylobacter, another very common form of gastroenteritis, the organisms are not normally spread that easily. A person could feasibly work on low-risk activity whilst convalescing from the illness.

**Q67 What is the most common source of infection from a food handler?**

A There are a number of common sources of potential infections including the nose, mouth, skin, hair in the case of Staphylococcus aureus, and the gut in the case of Salmonella, Escherichia coli and many other food poisoning organisms. The most common vehicle, however, is the hands. Whilst they are touching various parts of the body, either by habit or necessity, they transfer organisms via the fingertips and fingernails to foods and food contact surfaces.

**Q68 What risk is there from wearing normal clothing while handling food?**

A There are a number of risks from foreign material including buttons, threads, hairs, other fibres, etc and from bacteria including Staphylococcus, Salmonella, Clostridium perfringens and Escherichia coli. It should be noted, however, that whilst the risks are apparent they are small. Nevertheless, there is a legal requirement under the **Food Safety (General Food Hygiene) Regulations 1995** for food handlers to wear particular types of overclothing while they are carrying out food handling activities.

**Q69 Why should head coverings be worn in a food area?**

A Head coverings serve two useful purposes.

- They prevent hairs and dandruff falling from the head onto clothing and food contact surfaces or food itself (we lose an average 50 hairs each day).
- They restrict the habit of scratching the head which may transfer Staphylococcus organisms onto the fingers and consequently onto food.

Whilst the **Food Safety (General Food Hygiene) Regulations 1995** do not specify hats or head coverings, they do state that "suitable protective overclothing shall be worn" by food handlers. Most enforcement officers would view this as a requirement for head coverings.

**Q70 Why should I not smoke in and around food rooms and can I smoke a pipe?**

A It is illegal to smoke in food rooms according to the **Food Safety (General Food Hygiene) Regulations 1995**; there is a danger that bacteria, particularly Staphylococcus aureus, will be passed from the mouth onto fingers and onto food whilst smoking. There is a lesser risk with pipes but the pipe can be termed a hand-contact surface and the constant contact with "foamite" may provide a vehicle for bacteria to be transferred.

The ash and tobacco is also a foreign material risk.

**Q71 Is there a definitive list of when staff should wash their hands?**

A No. However, it should be remembered that hand washing is the most important part of personal hygiene practice and staff should wash their hands whenever there is a risk of contamination to the next job they are undertaking. Staff should wash their hands after all of the following (this list is by no means exhaustive):

- upon entering the food premises
- after using the toilet

- after smoking and eating
- after sneezing
- after handling refuse
- between handling raw and cooked foods
- after cleaning operations and handling cleaning chemicals
- after handling cash.

The general rule should be to wash hands whenever there is a potential risk of contamination to the next process being undertaken.

**Q72 What is the best form of hand-drying facility for a catering unit?**

A Probably paper towels. However, there are advantages and disadvantages with all systems. Retractable cloth towels can run out at inopportune times and often require replenishment by a contractor, so they may not be as reliable as one would wish. Air hand-dryers, whilst they appear to be ideal, are rarely used properly by busy catering staff. There is insufficient time in a busy catering business for drying of hands by this method. It is entirely possible that viral gastroenteritis outbreaks could be compounded by the use of air hand-dryers. Moist or wet hands are an extreme food safety risk and viruses can persist without the need or possibility of multiplication. Low infective doses can cause cases.

Paper towels are easily replenished and stocks can be readily available on site.

**Q73 Is there any food safety advantage to my staff wearing disposable gloves while handling high-risk foods?**

A Disposable gloves provide a false sense of security to the wearer and prevent frequent hand washing. Cross-contamination from the person or from objects touched with the plastic gloves can still occur to food. Nevertheless, with adequate supervision and readily available supplies of gloves there may be opportunities to limit some potential contaminants, particularly Staphylococcus aureus. Certainly food manufacturers, flight caterers, some contract caterers and other high-risk industries make use of such protective gloves.

**Q74 When do food handlers have to report infections?**

A Under the **Food Safety (General Food Hygiene) Regulations 1995**, food handlers must report any infection which may be transmitted through food. This could include gastroenteritis or skin infections.

**Q75 Is it necessary to provide hand-washing facilities at temporary outdoor barbecues?**

A They would certainly be extremely advantageous but it may be possible to provide bactericidal hand-wipes as an alternative. Views on this subject vary; it can depend on your EHO's personal opinion whether they think washing facilities are a necessity or not.

# PESTS

**Q76 I have a problem with flies within my catering business. What are the practical solutions?**

A All businesses will be affected by a few flies, particularly in the summer months, but large numbers of flies are often caused by unsatisfactory hygiene conditions within the kitchen. The following measures should help to reduce the nuisance.

- General hygiene within the kitchen, including floor cleaning, removal of refuse, lids to bins and thorough cleaning throughout.
- Regular cleaning of bins and skips, weekly if possible, after collection has been undertaken. More regular collection would be advantageous. Most flies come from outside areas, particularly refuse bins and skips.
- Thorough daily cleaning of outside areas, hosing down of yards, drains, etc.
- Fly screening to doors and windows, particularly where kitchens back onto refuse areas and yards.
- Keeping refuse stored within clean hygienic fly-proofed housings within the yard.
- Checking of all foods stored within catering areas on a regular basis to ensure that adequate stock rotation is occurring and attraction of flies is prevented.
- Removal of clutter from yard areas, bottle stores, etc.

**Q77 Where are electronic fly-killing units best sited?**

A They should be located in dark areas of the preparation rooms and left switched on throughout the night. They may, however, cause contamination to food and utensils including pans and preparation surfaces if the units are located above these areas as dead insects may fall onto the equipment or surfaces. Doorways, corridors and open wall spaces are the best places to site them in order to avoid this risk.

**Q78 Are electronic fly-killing units a necessary requirement in all food areas?**

A They have been shown not to be effective against all types of flying insects as many are not attracted to the ultraviolet light. Perhaps only 20% of insects will be destroyed by this method. The emphasis should be on preventing flies from entering the premises rather than attempting to eliminate them once they are present, which could potentially cause contamination.

**Q79 A number of my customers have noticed small black flies hovering around the bar areas. What are they and how may they be eliminated?**

A These are fruit flies (Drosophila) and they are most common in areas where perished or rotten food is present. The main precautions to prevent the flies appearing in the bar area are as follows.

- Cleanliness with scrupulous attention to corners.
- Regular removal of refuse.
- Any perished food stocks should be immediately removed.
- Empty bottles should not be stored in food areas.
- Regular cleaning of bins, bottle skips and bottle cap holders should be undertaken.
- Corners and edges of shelves should be checked and regularly cleaned.
- Post-mix rooms should be thoroughly cleaned and spillages immediately removed.

**Q80 Can a cockroach infestation be fully eliminated from a food premises?**

A It is extremely difficult to achieve total elimination of such insect pests within a food business. Fumigation is one of the only known methods and this would involve the complete sealing of the whole building and use of toxic gases which can seep into every crack and crevice. This is not always a practical proposition. Good quality and thorough pest control measures can have a dramatic effect but often if such areas as ducting, boxings in, etc are neglected it is possible that the insects will re-emerge. The treatment should be repeated about six weeks after the initial treatment to destroy any recently emerged cockroach nymphs. The choice of insecticide is also important with high-residual substances used in inaccessible areas.

**Q81 I believe that my outside areas are infested with rats. What are the most common signs of infestation and possible sources?**

A Common signs include the following.

- Burrows — particularly in earth banks around broken drainage, in amongst rubble, etc.
- Trails — they follow the same line to and from and around the premises.
- Smears and hairs around pipes and holes in the structure — they leave greasy marks and hairs around holes.
- Smell — there is a characteristic rodent smell in confined spaces.
- Droppings — these can be left in and around burrows, confined areas, sub-floors, dead spaces.
- Sightings — rats are mainly nocturnal and a night watch may be necessary to confirm suspicions.

All rodents are extremely destructive. They can chew through timber, lead and plastic providing they can get a hold. They will damage drainage, pipework and doors to gain access to food areas. Drains are the usual habitat of brown rats and they will often gain access to the surface through broken or defective drainage. Access to the building can also be via doors, broken windows, gaps and holes in brickwork or by service conduits including electricity, water and gas. They often emerge at the back of electricity board equipment within the premises or perhaps in the roof space, having gained access through the cavity.

**Q82 I believe my pest control operator is feeding the rodents rather than trying to get rid of them. What should I do? The infestation persists.**

A There are a number of reasons for this which include the following.

- The pest control operator may not be conducting his or her activities to the required standards, eg the baits may be old and stale and perhaps unappetising!

- Baits may be in the wrong places — they should be in concealed areas out of sight. Rodents do not like to be disturbed or obviously visible!
- Baits may be of insufficient strength or incorrect consistency.
- There may be resistance to the bait in use. Warfarin is the most common anticoagulant poison used and some resistance to it has built up amongst rat populations in certain parts of the country. In such circumstances it is necessary to change the type of anticoagulant poison used.

**Q83 What sort of poisons are available for killing rodents and can I carry out the work myself?**

A It is not advisable to carry out pest control in catering premises on a self-help basis; this is best left to a recognised pest control contractor. A considerable amount of training and skill is needed and baits may be extremely hazardous depending on which type is used.

There are three main types of pest bait available.

- Acute poisons — these are sometimes used in sewers and areas where the public cannot gain easy admission. They are extremely toxic and only one dose would be necessary.
- Chronic poisons — these include Warfarin and Difacoum. They require multi-takes by the rodent and are generally anticoagulant in nature, ie they prevent clotting of blood. The rodent dies from internal haemorrhage.
- Narcotic — these baits are usually used for birds. Users will need to be licensed by the Ministry of Agriculture, Fisheries and Food. These poisons are used in conjunction with a seed or meal base and the birds are narcotised, fall asleep, and are then collected and humanely destroyed and disposed of.

**Q84 I have noticed a rather horrible odour in and around the public rooms in my unit. What is it likely to be and what is the solution?**

A It is highly likely that a dead rodent or rodents have caused this odour. Anticoagulant baits act over a sustained period of time which allows the rodent to escape from the area in which it consumed the bait. Rats and mice can often end up under floors or staging, in cavities, ducting, trunkings, etc where they begin to decay with a most foul odour. It will be necessary to locate the dead rodent and remove it. The smell will then quickly disappear. This can take quite some time and effort. It is possible to mask the smell until the rodent is fully decayed but this is not a good option under the circumstances. If you allow this to happen be ready for the presence of a few flies around the premises!

**Q85 What is the difference between food pest and incidental pest?**

A The food pests include rats, mice, cockroaches, flies (blue bottles, house flies), larvae beetle, weevils, mites, flour moths, etc. These all have one thing in common, ie they are interested in gaining access to premises in order to search out our food. They can cause considerable damage, reducing and spoiling food stocks and causing a continued infestation until action is taken.

Incidental pests include garden beetles, crickets, wasps and bees, black jacks, earwigs, large moths, crane flies, wood lice and rabbits. While these pests are often infuriating and most objectionable they are not particularly after our food but merely wander into our food areas to cause nuisance. Some pests, including wood lice and earwigs, often enjoy damp conditions. If these conditions could be removed then the pests would also be reduced. They all may cause a foreign material risk to food.

**Q86 How can I get rid of birds from my kitchen?**

A From time to time, birds may enter premises, particularly if there are large galleried canteens with kitchens attached. They are attracted by food residues and spillages to outside bin areas initially, and may try to find richer pickings inside. The main emphasis should be on prevention; this may include mist netting over windows and protection of refuse areas outside. Certainly no member of staff should encourage birds, particularly pigeons, by leaving food out for them. All such creatures are food pests and carry harmful bacteria including Campylobacter and Salmonella species.

**Note:** It is illegal to kill wild birds. Many of them are protected, even some of the more common varieties such as starlings, sparrows and magpies. Pigeons can be controlled only by licensed contractors under the direction of the Ministry of Agriculture, Fisheries and Food.

**Q87 My EHO has requested that I fit fly screens to all my kitchen windows. Do I really have to go to the expense?**

A It depends. If your EHO feels that there is a risk of pest infestation through the windows of your kitchen, then you are required to fit fly screens. However, if you are not affected by flying insects there is no requirement. You should clarify the situation with your EHO and ask them to justify the necessity for such screens. It is of course good practice to have screens fitted to any opening windows in your kitchen.

**Q88 My EHO has said that all the waste bins in my kitchen must be kept lidded. Is this really a practical proposition when they are constantly in use throughout the day?**

A No. There is no requirement for lids to be fitted to containers used for the temporary storage of waste in food preparation areas. Lids are a potential source of contamination. However, any receptacle used for the storage of waste awaiting collection by the refuse collectors should have a lid.

# CATERING DESIGN

**Q89 What are the most important aspects of design for a kitchen?**

A The **Food Safety (General Food Hygiene) Regulations 1995** form the basis of design criteria for kitchens and must be complied with in the interests of food hygiene. They can be summarised as follows.

- Cleanliness — it is necessary to have readily cleansable surfaces which are all easily accessible. Smooth walls, floors, ceilings without gaps or awkward corners are necessary. All equipment should be on wheels with flexible couplings to assist cleanliness.
- Food handling — the environment of the kitchen should be as cool as practicable with good ventilation to reduce the risk of increasing food temperatures. Consideration should be given to ergonomic design to ensure that cross-contamination between raw and cooked preparation work is reduced. It is important that refrigeration is located conveniently accessible to workstations and food storage facilities are also conveniently accessible to avoid ad hoc storage within the kitchen.
- Maintenance — it is important that all surfaces are durable and protected against damage. Metal edging strips at the corners of surfaces and along wall surfaces in corridors can assist in this respect.
- Health and safety — choice of non-slip surfaces, good positioning of dangerous equipment and care with electricity and chemical storage are vital with respect to design.
- Pest control — it is important that access is prevented for pests, eg measures such as fly screens, door screens, elimination of dead spaces should be adopted as much as is practicable and refuse storage measures should be strictly adhered to.

**Q90 What are good tips to ensure my kitchen can be easily and effectively cleaned?**

A Where to begin! The first and most basic tip is to ensure that your kitchen is well designed and maintained. It is a lot easier to clean a kitchen with smooth non-absorbent surfaces, no hidden nooks and crannies, easily movable equipment and good work flows. The easier you make the job, the more likely it will be done. Second, "clean as you go"; don't leave all the cleaning until the end of the day, as this is when short cuts are taken. You should try to introduce a food safety culture where your staff automatically carry out such tasks as cleaning without being asked. Training is essential to help achieve this. Third, cleaning schedules (outlining what is to be cleaned, when and by whom) provide an excellent management tool to ensure that cleaning is being carried out. Finally, you must ensure that you have the right tools and cleaning materials for the job and that staff are fully trained on how to use them.

**Q91 I am considering a new floor for my kitchen. What is the best surface recommended?**

A There are a number of choices which include ceramic tiles, linoleum type surfaces and resin floors. However, ceramic tiles laid with fine epoxy resin grouting would be the most durable surface. Both resin and vinyl-type surfaces tend to be more easily damaged by heat or mechanical impact. Light colours should always be the norm in catering areas — it is necessary to see the dirt rather than hide it.

**Q92 How can I ensure that the requirements for floors are met when they have to be non-slip surfaces for health and safety purposes, yet cleansable with respect to food hygiene?**

A This is probably one of the most difficult compromises to be made in kitchens. Wet floors account for one third of all accidents in kitchens. However, surfaces which are smooth, impervious and capable of being cleaned are not always particularly safe. Where possible, floor surfaces should be selected with a greater slip resistance; often these will incorporate a Carborundum finish. If possible, such surfaces should only be used in walkways as they can be difficult to keep clean, particularly ceramic tiled surfaces. Linoleum-type surfaces tend to be more easily cleaned.

**Q93 I have been recommended to have a grease trap installed within the catering area. Will this cause problems?**

A Certainly it is not advisable to have a grease trap installed within the kitchen area, but it may be a practical solution external to the kitchen where it can be easily attended to with regard to maintenance, servicing, etc. Emphasis, however, should be placed on elimination of grease from drains. No food waste should be discharged into drainage including oil, grease, etc. Pans should be fully scraped out prior to being washed. Skimming of sinks after washing of greasy pans is advisable. Use of enzymes which digest grease should be considered.

**Q94 Whatever happened to kitchen drains? We seemed so much better off with them.**

A Floor drains tend not to be a design feature of new kitchens due to the problems of cleanliness that can arise through poor hygiene management. They are also a potential harbourage for pests. However, if this type of drain is cleaned regularly as part of a written cleaning schedule and is provided with grids, there is no reason why it cannot continue to be used.

# FOOD PREPARATION

**Q95 Why are wooden utensils and cutting boards no longer satisfactory for food handling? I have heard that polypropylene scratches easily and contains more bacteria than wood.**

A Essentially, wooden equipment could be considered to be illegal under the **Food Safety (General Food Hygiene) Regulations 1995** which states that all equipment that comes in contact with food shall be clean, non-toxic, impervious and capable of being kept clean. Wood is not a substance which would be satisfactory in this respect and a move to more hygienic polypropylene equipment is advised. However, scratched or scored polypropylene is certainly not hygienic as such scratches may harbour bacteria. It should be remembered that polypropylene equipment will not last forever and perhaps has a life of 3–6 months before it is in a condition that is no longer capable of being cleaned. It should then be replaced. It is possible that thicker boards could be planed to a smooth surface again but this is not generally a do-it-yourself operation. Small equipment, such as cutting boards and food utensils, should be replaced regularly and an adequate budget should be available for this purpose in all catering businesses.

**Q96 How can I prevent cross-contamination within my kitchen?**

A There are usually two events which need to happen before food poisoning can occur:

- contamination with pathogenic organisms of food which is ready to eat without further preparation, and
- incubation of those bacteria to produce large numbers of bacteria or their toxins.

With this in mind, cross-contamination with low-risk foods (ie those not containing protein or foods which are to be further prepared) is not likely to be that significant. However, one should not rely on the process of heating to act as the final food hygiene measure to prevent food poisoning. There are a number of options to prevent cross-contamination.

- Segregation of areas within the kitchen — this is sometimes impractical in small areas. However, raw meat, fish and vegetables could be kept out of main cooking areas until they are needed and prepared in separate areas of the kitchen.
- Segregation by time — it would be better to prepare finished foods first, eg sandwiches and buffets, rather than do the raw preparation work first.
- Segregated food handlers — transfer of bacteria on hands, clothing, etc can be a significant risk. If certain workers can be assigned to all raw preparation work and others to finished foods then this would help to eliminate the risk. However, this may not always be possible in some catering operations. Disposable aprons are a further option.
- Reduction of raw products entering the premises — certain operations lend themselves to ready prepared foods, prepared sweets and cakes, and vegetables can be ready peeled, meats for cold buffets can be ready cooked — such supplies will all be a considerable help and take much of the labour and effort out of catering. It can, however, take out some of the quality if purchasing decisions are poor.
- Colour-coding of knives, cutting boards, food utensils, containers, mops, trays, sink areas, etc. It will then be obvious to a supervisor or chef that the wrong knife, etc is being used for a particular food, allowing adequate supervision to be maintained. This is a great advantage in preventing contamination but can be abused and is no substitute for effective regular cleaning of all equipment after use.
- Sanitising after raw preparation work — this is probably the easiest and most reliable method of preventing cross-contamination. All equipment, including slicers, mixers, cutting boards, table tops, knives, etc that come into contact with food should be thoroughly sanitised after use before the next activity. Generally, a fast-acting chlorine-based sanitiser is recommended so that the food handler can get on with the next job expeditiously.

Thinking on this concept of contamination and incubation has recently been modified. In the past, temperature control has been seen as the cure for all ills. There was less emphasis on the way the food was handled because refrigeration would ensure that any bugs would not multiply to a level that would cause food poisoning. With the events of Lanarkshire we know now that this approach is not acceptable. Food-borne infections (such as E.coli 0157 and Campylobacter) do not require a period of time at ambient temperature to cause illness because the infective dose is small. For instance, to contract Salmonella food poisoning you would have to consume about 6 million organisms — for E.coli 0157 and Campylobacter it could be as few as 10–100 organisms. Therefore, prevention of contamination is of the utmost importance. The Pennington report, which was published following the outbreak of E.coli poisoning in Lanarkshire, recommends increasing legal requirements for separating high-risk foods from contamination (such as providing separate counters for cooked and raw meat). It is likely that new laws will be passed to reflect this advice.

**Q97 Why is the cooling of food so vitally important to food hygiene?**

A Food in the danger zone of 5–63°C has the capability of multiplying micro-organisms. Certain bacteria are not destroyed by the heat of cooking and form spores which are a mechanism of survival for certain bacteria. When the food begins to cool at the end of the cooking process and the temperature falls back into the danger zone below 63°C, the spores "germinate" and vegetative bacteria (ie which are live and capable of reproduction) are then again available to multiply and potentially cause food poisoning. The effective cooling of foods is perhaps the most important process in food hygiene besides that of avoidance of contamination. It can be carried out in a number of ways.

- Initially reducing the volume and mass of food to be cooked, particularly meats like large pork/beef joints or turkeys. Ideally 2.7kg or 6lb joints should be the largest cooked.
- Using a blast chiller which will cool most foods within 1.5 hours to below 3°C.
- Removing meat and other foods from the juices and placing on cool, clean trays in a cool part of the kitchen.
- Using ice with vegetables.
- Reducing the volumes of liquid dishes into trays with a larger surface area.
- Using cold water and ice around cooking pots within food preparation sinks.

**Q98 Does all food have to be defrosted before it is cooked?**

A No. Generally you should follow the manufacturer's advice. Some products (such as beefburgers) can be cooked direct from the freezer. However, with larger items such as poultry, if they are not properly defrosted the usual cooking time will be insufficient to raise the core temperature of the food to a level where pathogenic bacteria are killed.

**Q99 My refrigerator is a long way from the hot kitchen. How long can I keep raw meat and fish out before it must be cooked?**

A Although raw meat carries pathogenic bacteria which will multiply in the hot kitchen, cooking ensures that any bacteria will be killed off (as long as it is done properly). As such, there are no requirements regarding the temperature control of raw meat. However, it is good practice to keep it refrigerated for as long as possible. Fish follow the same rule for the most part. However, care must be taken with oily fish such as tuna or mackerel (known as "scombroids"). If the raw fish is stored at above 4°C, decomposition will produce a toxin which can cause food poisoning (Scombrotoxic food poisoning). Care must also be taken with smoked and cured fish which does not require cooking. As a general rule, do not remove anything from the fridge unless you need it and put it away when you've finished with it.

**Q100 Why should pot plants not be allowed in food preparation or service areas?**

A Whilst such decorative plants add colour and interest to a restaurant area, they should not be placed in food preparation areas as they may provide contamination of food. There are a number of ways in which this may occur, as follows.

- Leaves, flower petals, decaying stems and other such material may provide a foreign material risk to food.
- Plants often attract flying insects, beetles and other such pests which, while not actually being food pests, may nevertheless also contaminate foods.

- The soil or growth media can be spilt on food; it may be dislodged through accident or during watering and bacteria including Listeria or Clostridium perfringens may be a risk to food in preparation.

It may be possible to allow dried flowers and other such basket displays at servery areas. This is particularly evident at motorway services. Care must be taken, however, to ensure that such materials do not contaminate salad displays and other unprotected food. They must be carefully managed and positioned to ensure that this does not occur. Above all they should not be allowed to get dusty with accumulations of spiders' webs — this would not be a substitute for fly control!

**Q101 How can I ensure the safe washing of fruits and salad items so that they are ready for consumption by the consumer?**

A Generally these items are by no means high risk. However, a small number of food-borne infections can cause a risk to the consumer, including E.coli, Campylobacter, Dysentery and Viral Gastroenteritis. In the case of more classic food poisoning organisms, the risks presented by all such foods may be increased if salad items are to be combined with high-risk foods, eg fish, meat or eggs, perhaps for sandwiches and buffets, etc.

All such food products should be washed in a clean bowl or sink which has been properly sanitised and they should be allowed to soak in a weak sterile solution in the order of 10/20 parts per million; if the concentration is any higher than this, destruction of the vegetable matter may occur resulting in "off" taints and flavours. The solution is made up with sterilising tablets which are commercially available for such use. The solution can be tested with test papers to ensure there is sufficient strength.

**Q102 Can sanitisers be used for washing salad and fruit items as well as to disinfect food contact surfaces?**

A Whilst all sanitisers should be food safe, they are not recommended for the washing of such foods. They contain other chemicals, often detergents, which may be irritating to the mucous membranes or perhaps the intestines.

**Q103 What special precautions do I have to undertake when carrying out catering outdoors?**

A Such catering is normally carried out in the summer months when ambient temperatures are generally much higher, therefore there is a risk from finished food temperatures rising and the consequential multiplication of harmful bacteria.

Flies and other insects can also be a problem with easy transfer of micro-organisms from outdoor toilet facilities onto food. The environment may also produce a risk of food contamination, particularly from the ground and also airborne dusts and debris. It is important, therefore, that additional precautions are taken to avoid such contamination. Considerable risks are created by the use of part-time staff who perhaps are only required for short periods and may not have a sufficient knowledge of food hygiene. This also requires careful consideration before planning such events. Organisers must ensure there is adequate refrigeration of all foods prior to preparation and service, and provide for surfaces which can be easily cleaned for the duration of the event. Temporary floors, walls, etc can be created at low cost. Washing-up sinks and wash-hand basins will be needed and with a little good planning they can be supplied with hot water, soap and towels.

**Q104 Why do some pre-prepared sandwiches have a lot of information on the packaging while others have none? As a caterer, do I have to label the sandwiches that I prepare?**

A Labelling of food is controlled by the **Food Labelling Regulations 1996**. Generally food must be labelled with the following information:

- the name of the food
- a list of ingredients
- an appropriate durability indication (ie "use by" or "best before" date)
- any special storage instructions (eg "refrigerate after opening")
- the name and address of the manufacturer.

However, there is an exemption for food which is "pre-packed for direct sale", which means any food which is packed on the same premises as it is sold on. Therefore, as long as you are preparing the sandwiches yourself for sale on your premises, you do not have to provide any labelling on the sandwiches. Generally, sandwiches that have a large amount of information on their packaging have been prepared "off-site".

# COOKING AND REHEATING

**Q105 What are the main hazards in using a microwave for cooking and how can I overcome them?**

A There are several food safety hazards to consider. First, there is a tendency these days to use microwaves for the primary cooking of raw food and defrosting. This then provides a risk of cross-contamination if the more traditional use of reheating cooked food is undertaken later. Ideally, separate microwaves should be considered. Second, there is a risk of "cool spots" in dense foods and therefore adequate reheating and monitoring with a probe thermometer is recommended.

**Q106 Without using a probe thermometer how can I tell if food is thoroughly cooked?**

A Caterers should know the signs and tests which establish whether food is properly cooked. Much of it is down to experience and training and this is an increasingly important issue with regard to hazard analysis. Signs include the tightening of meat sinews which are visually and texturally apparent. Colour change and clear juices are other signs which indicate cooked meat. Tests depend on the type of dish being prepared but if, for example, you are able to lift a piece of chuck beef in a sauce with a small knife vertically placed in it, there is the good likelihood that the sinews of the meat have tightened up and that it is cooked through. A good test for skewered meat kebab-style is to shake it to see if there is any movement. A "wobble" of the piece of meat would indicate that gelatinous uncooked conditions still exist, in other words it needs a bit more cooking before service. The use of a probe thermometer is, however, always recommended to validate the above.

**Q107 Why is there a need to cook burgers thoroughly when beef can be eaten rare?**

A Diced/minced meat is inherently more prone to contamination as it is processed through mechanical equipment and also it may not be the best cut of meat (contamination can then be found in the centre of the burger). E.coli, Salmonella, Campylobacter and Clostridium perfringens are all possibilities from diced meat and only thorough cooking until juices run clear will prevent the potential of food poisoning from burgers. Contamination of a joint of beef is usually on the surface. Serving rare will still ensure the surface is subjected to a high enough temperature to kill the majority of bacteria, even if the inside is still bloody.

**Q108 Is there any health risk in producing rare beef and steaks for my customers?**

A Rare beef and steaks are not thoroughly cooked and there is a potential (though extremely small) health risk. Meat only browns when it reaches 65°C to 70°C — this is a sufficient temperature to kill bacteria. Rare meats may have reached, at best, 50°C or 55°C — which would not have killed pathogenic bacteria. However, it is highly unlikely that the centre of a steak or (non-rolled) joint would be contaminated with pathogenic bacteria if freshly prepared and freshly cooked. Contamination is usually confined to the outside of the meat which has been cooked and possibly contaminated by contact with a knife, cutting board or chopping block. However, these areas are usually cauterised and reach a temperature which will kill any bacteria upon them

Rare beefburgers and sausages are a different proposition. Diced meat is highly contaminated because it has a large surface area that has been through a mincer which is itself highly contaminated. There is also a risk involved with steak tartare and rolled joints. Serving these foods raw is extremely dangerous. E.coli 0157 is a particularly nasty organism which has seen a considerable rise in numbers, often due to undercooked beef and lamb products. Tapeworm cysts are another significant (but thankfully rare) occurrence in the UK. One should expect that the meat inspector would cut these out. Thorough cooking would eliminate such cysts but this would not occur in very rare steaks, so there is still a small risk.

Rolled, boned joints may be similarly contaminated through contact with equipment and therefore may be hazardous if they are under-cooked.

**Q109 I often cook joints of meat on one day, then cool them down and reheat the next day. How long can I hold each food and to what temperature should I reheat it?**

A The **Food Safety (Temperature Control) Regulations 1995** require that hot food is maintained at above 63°C with an exemption of two hours for service and display. Cooling of the joint should be carried out as quickly as possible and preferably in a blast chiller. If this is not available, the joint should be cool enough to go in the fridge in 90 minutes. To help achieve this, ensure that joints of meat are kept as small as possible (less than 2.5 kg). The meat should then be stored at below 5°C until required. Reheating should aim to achieve a core temperature of 82°C to ensure that any pathogens are killed.

**Q110 What is the difference between the core temperature of food when it is cooked and the holding temperature of food during service? Why is there such a difference?**

A There is a need to cook food to a high enough temperature in order to destroy pathogenic micro-organisms and make the food palatable to eat. With chicken and pork this is considered to be about 82°C. With beef, other than a rolled boned joint, the temperature could be as low as 55°C in practice, which would have the similar effect but leave the meat rather rare.

It takes a hot oven and considerable time, depending on the weight and density of the meat, to ensure the whole of the meat achieves these core temperatures. The surface is likely to heat up well above the core temperature and reach perhaps 95°C in the case of poultry, whilst the inside attains only 82°C. Once these core temperatures have been achieved it is then satisfactory to hold the temperature at about 63°C in a hot cupboard or on a hot tray under hot lamps on a servery or perhaps a carvery. The aim at this stage is to have a high enough temperature to ensure that any spore-producing bacteria do not come within the danger zone (ie 5–63°C) where the spores may germinate and produce vegetative (ie living) bacteria again. It is a further aim that the meat should not carry on cooking as this will reduce its quality, increase its toughness and remove moisture; 63°C is considered an adequate temperature for these purposes as well.

**Q111 Can I be sure that reheating pre-cooked food will make it safe if it has been at room temperature for a while?**

A No. There are a number of pathogenic bacteria that can cause illness despite thorough reheating. Clostridium perfringens is an anaerobic bacterium that is associated with meat, stews and gravy. It is capable of forming spores that can survive cooking. If the product being cooked is allowed to cool slowly, the spores germinate and multiply on the food. Reheating may be insufficient to kill the bacteria which can then cause food poisoning. Bacillus cereus and Staphylococcus aureus are two pathogenic bacteria that produce a toxin on the food if allowed to multiply at ambient temperatures. These toxins are able to withstand very high temperatures and therefore reheating will not prevent the risk of food poisoning. Remember food should be cooled as quickly as possible and reheated to a minimum of 82°C.

**Q112 What are the main foreign material risks within the kitchen?**

A Sources of foreign material risk can be put into six main groups.

- Raw products for processing — there may be inherent risks in quite natural constituents of some foods, eg shells, stones, bones, stalks, etc.
- Packaging — if packaging becomes dislodged it may be incorporated into food from an early stage in processing, eg wood splinters, glass, paper, cardboard, string, staples, etc. This is a particular problem when boxes and bags of food are decanted in the kitchen rather than in a separate area.
- Personnel — eg hairs, fingernails, buttons, pens, combs, threads.
- Pests — eg dead bodies of insects, legs, wings, droppings, hairs.
- Plant and equipment — eg nuts, bolts, flaking paint, pieces of perspex, guarding, sheared metal pieces.
- Premises — eg flaking paint, plaster, broken tiles, glass from shattered windows or lighting units.

**Q113 How can risks from foreign matter be reduced?**

A Risks from foreign matter can be reduced by the following.

- Taking care with the processing chain is important. Measures should be introduced to ensure quality control of food to be processed and that the best source of supply is used.
- Ensuring that packaging is removed at an early stage and not brought into kitchens.
- Requiring high standards of personal hygiene amongst staff.
- Ensuring the maintenance of kitchen structure and equipment.
- Controlling pests.
- Good standards of cleaning — clean as you go! (See Q135.)

**Q114 I have heard much about keeping food reasonably cool while it is being prepared. What advice is there to ensure this is undertaken?**

A Being well organised with regard to preparation of the various elements of a menu is vital. A high-risk food for preparation should only be brought out when it is anticipated that time is available to work on that particular food.

There is a need for both bulk and localised refrigeration within catering areas. The localised area, perhaps an under-counter refrigerator, is useful for ingredients and work in progress. The bulk refrigerator should only be used for raw or prepared products and door openings can be limited to a minimum. There is a need to restore food temperatures after work on food has been completed. This could be undertaken in a large cold room or perhaps a chiller, but a blast chiller can also be used for this purpose if available.

High-risk foods including cooked meats, cream, gravy, meat stocks, quiches, pastries, egg dishes, mayonnaise, etc should all be kept as cold as possible during preparation. Introducing any energy into food, eg by whisking, mixing or slicing will raise the temperature. Increasing the surface area of the food will allow the ambient temperature of the kitchen and preparation areas which are in contact with food to lift up its temperatures. The best advice is as follows.

- Work on small batches of food at a time.
- Do any low-risk operations first, eg buttering of bread for sandwiches.
- Slice cooked meats or whisk cream and then restore its temperature in a chiller before using it.

- Produce food in small batches and refrigerate each batch after it has been produced.
- Keep food under refrigeration as long as is practicable before service.
- Do not undertake high-risk food activities in hot areas. Use cooler larder areas.
- Consider the use of cold surfaces, eg marble or, if available, chilled wells within the kitchen for preparation.
- Raw food (such as fish or pieces of meat or chicken) can be kept in a perforated tray on a bed of ice prior to cooking.

**Q115 Does blast chilling have a role to play in small catering establishments or is it merely a high-volume mass production tool?**

A Blast chilling equipment is certainly a valuable addition in terms of hygiene within any catering business. It should certainly not be confined to just high-volume businesses. Small commercial blast chillers which can undertake the chilling of 30–50lbs of food or less within 1.5 hours are available from a number of suppliers and they have many uses:

- blast chilling of cooked food to below 3°C when it can be stored within a refrigerator
- restoring of temperatures of foods in preparation, eg cream, sandwich mixes such as tuna mayonnaise
- chilling of eggs and egg dishes
- pre-chilling of foods to be put on ambient buffet displays after preparation
- chilling of food which was intended for service but which has not been sold and is therefore intended for re-service
- ingredients used to make up foods
- chilling of "overproduction".

The basic concept of temperature control is an extremely important issue and if this concept was in the mind of every caterer there would certainly be less risk of food poisoning within the industry.

**Q116 I am considering purchasing a vacuum-packing machine for my catering business as I understand the life of foods can be made considerably longer. Are there any risks from using such equipment?**

A Certainly the exclusion of air from products will prevent certain bacteria from multiplying and therefore the shelf-life of food can be improved. Vacuum-packing alone, however, is extremely dangerous and all foods should be stored under refrigeration below 3°C. Only raw foods which are to be further prepared and cooked, including steaks, poultry and perhaps vegetables should be vacuum-packed. Cooked foods should not be vacuum-packed in catering premises as the hygiene standards cannot be guaranteed and the degree of control needed is difficult to achieve. All vacuum-packed food should be date coded with the date on which it was packed and the shelf-life should generally be kept to below five days including the date of packing and date of use. This is in accordance with the cook-chill guidelines. Whilst longer shelf-lives are possible there are dangers.

The main risk of vacuum-packing food is that whilst aerobic (oxygen-loving) bacteria are prevented from growth, certain anaerobic bacteria may grow in profusion once the air has been excluded. One particularly serious bacterium would be Clostridium botulinum or the disease of botulism. This is a deadly disease caused by a toxin produced by the bacteria. Vacuum-packing and poor temperature control provide excellent conditions for growth, therefore it would not be wise to vacuum-pack foods in catering premises unless hygiene standards and control measures can be guaranteed. The risks outweigh the benefits.

**Q117 How can I ensure that chickens and other poultry are thoroughly cooked before service?**

A Whilst an experienced chef with a skewer who knows the performance of the cooking equipment would have little doubt in recognising when such foods are cooked, this is nevertheless an area of growing importance. Only a probe thermometer, properly calibrated and maintained using a sterilised wipe, can indicate when such foods are cooked. When poultry has reached 82°C it can be deemed to be cooked. If possible it should be served hot and not chilled and reheated.

**Q118 Is there any advantage in using the self-sanitising "Microban" cutting boards?**

A This is an interesting development that may have some value in the home where cutting boards are used generally less often and where soiling is lighter. For commercial use it is possible that staff might develop a false sense of security thinking they can work on both raw and cooked foods in quick succession. These products will not replace sensible colour coded systems and use of food safe chemical sanitisers.

**Q119 How can I ensure E.coli 0157 is prevented in my kitchen?**

A The key preventative actions are as follows.

- Purchase your meat from a reputable supplier.
- Ensure raw meat is kept separated during delivery, storage and preparation.
- Ensure good sanitising of food contact equipment, services and measures are taken to prevent cross contamination such as colour coded equipment and separate areas for raw meat.
- Thorough cooking is the key to preventing E.coli infection, particularly for meat products such as burgers, sausages and pies.
- Raw milk is a considerable risk and must be avoided by caterers (see also Q11).
- Good personal hygiene and handwashing.
- Thorough washing of salads and vegetables.

# CLEANING

**Q120 How many cleaning products do I need for an average kitchen?**

A It is impossible to say specifically what is required because it depends on the scale of the operation and activities undertaken. The following list provides a guide.

- Detergent for washing by hand — may be used for plates, cutlery, pots, pans, etc.
- Machine detergent — for dishwashers (not to be used for hand washing).
- A rinse aid — generally assists in removal of stains from finished crockery in a dishwasher.
- Sanitiser — for cleaning and destruction of micro-organisms on lightly soiled surfaces.
- Disinfectant — may not strictly be necessary but useful for drains, sink wastes, toilets, etc.
- Oven cleaner — a heavy duty degreaser for carbonised deposits on ovens and perhaps baking trays.
- Floor cleaning detergent — a low-foaming heavy-duty degreaser for floors.

**Q121 What is the difference between sanitisers and disinfectants and when should they be used?**

A A sanitiser is a chemical product which is able to both clean lightly soiled surfaces, having detergent properties, and destroy micro-organisms, reducing them to a level which is no longer harmful. A disinfectant does not have detergent properties and can only destroy micro-organisms. It should only be used after cleaning with a detergent has taken place.

Sanitisers have been developed in recent years to assist caterers with efficient effective cleaning only on lightly soiled surfaces such as preparation tables, cutting boards, etc.

**Q122 What is the best, most effective sanitising agent for my kitchens?**

A Chlorine-based sanitisers in the manufacturer's recommended dilution offer the most effective solution in a busy kitchen.

Chlorine has an almost immediate effect on bacteria and viruses preventing cross-contamination especially when surfaces and equipment need to be re-used again for preparation. Quaternary ammonia-based products — QUATS — can be used but they often have to be left in place for a contact time of 5–10 minutes to reduce micro-organisms to safe levels. Some manufacturers claim that they should be rinsed off but this process might result in re-contamination particularly if dirty cloths are used.

**Q123 Why are my detergents not successful against all grease and dirt found within the kitchen?**

A Generally, soiling is either organic or inorganic in nature. Organic soiling includes fats, grease, oils, blood, etc and inorganic soiling includes scales, milkstones, limescale, and uric acid stains in toilet areas.

Given different types of soil and degrees of soiling, detergents have to be formulated to deal with various situations. Generally, acid detergents, including the descalers, will break up and clean scales and inorganic types of soil while alkaline detergents will deal with the organic soils. It is important that the correct formulation and pH be used for different degrees of soiling of the different types, eg oven cleaners tend to be more powerful because they are more caustic than washing-up liquids intended for light grease on plates.

**Q124 A black line has built up around the edges of the toilet accommodation, bars and areas of the kitchen. Why does this occur and how can it be prevented?**

A This is typical within many premises. Even when it would appear that regular cleaning is being undertaken, deposits occur at the edges. There are two solutions:

- design — all wall/floor junctions should be coved within the catering premises to assist cleaning, and
- cleaning standards — these may be unsatisfactory because of a lack of energy in one or more of the following shown on the diagram below.

It is possible to reduce effort by ensuring that hot water and chemical concentration remains satisfactory for the task in hand. Should the water become cold and chemicals be used up then ineffective cleaning will occur — the dirt will simply be pushed to the edges of the floor where it will remain in deposits. These deposits should be scraped and special attention given to these areas in future. Training of staff with respect to chemical concentrations, hot water, etc is needed.

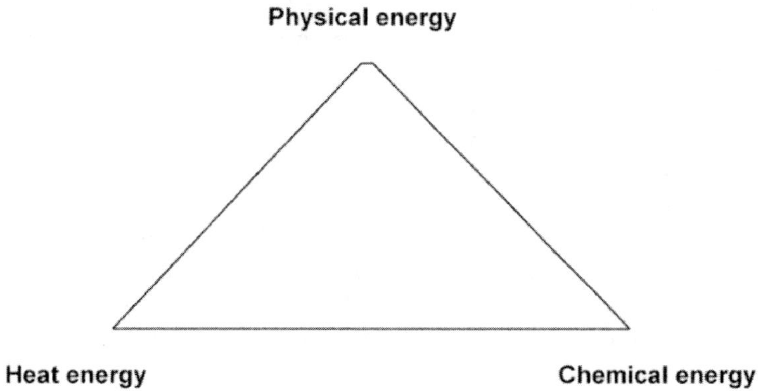


Another tip is to fill up the bucket with as much hot water as possible — it will stay hotter for longer that way!

**Q125 Are mops and buckets the most satisfactory method of floor cleaning within kitchen areas?**

A One might expect that the mop and bucket would have long been phased out of the kitchen hygiene system. However, they are still used extensively as the main method of floor cleaning. The concern is that in some circumstances they may be used in all areas (eg toilets, staff rooms, kitchens and sometimes the yard) and rather than cleaning surfaces, they simply transfer the micro-organisms from place to place. A colour coded system would help so that mops and buckets are designated for specific areas, particularly differentiating between toilets and food preparation areas. However, this does not in itself improve the use of this equipment which, given a poorly trained and motivated individual, may only serve to push dirt under tabling and into corners.

**ACTION PLAN FOR USE OF THE MOP AND BUCKET**

- Mops should be stored upright and allowed to dry out after use.
- The wash water should contain an adequate amount of detergent in extremely hot water. The bucket should be filled up.
- Efforts should be made to move as much tabling and equipment out of corners as possible before cleaning is undertaken.
- Some effort is required to mop the floor with the cleaning solution. The mop should be regularly turned through the bucket in order to transfer dirt into the bucket and retrieve fresh water for mopping.
- The temperature of the water will cool and the strength of the detergent will diminish while cleaning is in process so it is necessary to change the water frequently to ensure adequate standards of cleaning are maintained.
- Once the floor is clean a disinfectant solution should be mixed with hot water and the floor should receive a further treatment with this solution. Given good ventilation the floor should dry very quickly; drying is a good aid to destroying bacteria and other micro-organisms.

The above action plan certainly would ensure a high standard of floor cleaning and prevent build up of grease on the edges of the floor and in the grouting gaps between tiling.

**Note:** The floor is certainly not a high-risk area within catering premises and if time and resources are limited more effort should be put into sanitising of food contact surfaces.

**Q126 Is there any alternative to the mop and bucket for cleaning floors?**

A It is possible to use some form of floor scrubbing machine with water vacuum; this would certainly do a much better job than the mop and bucket. One of the difficulties, however, is the number of obstructions and awkward corners that occur in many kitchens. However, with more modern equipment on flexible hoses, this should not present a significant problem.

**Q127 What is the best method of ensuring sanitisation of food contact surfaces within kitchens?**

A Certainly this has always been a difficult question and it depends on how diligent the operator is. One method suggested by American sanitarians is the "three bucket" method. This involves three different coloured buckets; one containing a wash solution with hot water and detergent, another bucket containing hot water only, as a rinse solution, and a final bucket containing lukewarm water with a sanitising solution.

The procedure would be to wash the surface to be sanitised first, then rinse it to remove any debris and detergent, and then finally sanitise the surface once the first two processes have been undertaken. This is a very thorough method of sanitisation (disinfection).

Commercial sanitisers, however, would be adequate in light-soiling situations.

**Q128 How can I ensure that my sanitisers for food contact surfaces remain of adequate strength for their period of use?**

A This can prove rather difficult and it is important that if mixing to a solution is required, the correct ratios of sanitiser to water are satisfactory in the first place.

Powdered sanitisers can be used neat, via a shaker, onto surfaces and wiped with a clean cloth. Under such circumstances the strength is likely to be adequate providing recently delivered stocks are being used. Chlorine-based sanitisers are particularly easy to assess in terms of strength if they are mixed into solution, as test papers are available. This is not so easily done with other types of sanitiser, including quaternary ammonium compounds.

It is important that sanitisers in solution are only used for short periods and a new mixture is made at regular intervals. This would negate the need for testing.

**Q129 I do not have a dishwasher in my small catering unit. What is the best method of cleaning crockery?**

A The "two sink" method is the traditional method for this and the process is as follows.

- Step 1 — fill both sinks, one with hot water and detergent and the other with hot water, if possible at around 80°C or at 60°C with a disinfectant in it.
- Step 2 — plates and other articles to be washed should be properly scraped to remove as much debris as possible in order to keep the water as clean as possible.
- Step 3 — items should be washed thoroughly in the hot water and detergent to remove grease and debris.
- Step 4 — items should be placed within a clean wire basket vertically in order that they may drain, then placed within the second sink and left for around five minutes in order to allow a contact period in order to finish the sanitation process.
- Step 5 — items should then be removed and allowed to drain and "air dry" before stacking. There is little risk from using wiping cloths provided that they are clean, dry and regularly changed. Note that if the water remains reasonably clean and hot in both sinks then few, if any, stains will occur and there will be little need for drying with a cloth.

**Q130 I have problems with waste food in that nobody seems to wish to collect it these days. What is the best solution to this disposal problem?**

A Efforts should be made to reduce waste food volumes by taking care with portion control and stock rotation. There is no harm in mixing dry refuse and waste food and disposing of it through the normal refuse contracts. Problems are encountered when large containers of food waste, particularly wet liquid material, are placed into refuse bins. The ultimate solution is a waste disposal unit, but consent from the water authority would be needed. If all else fails it is possible to get such waste collected by a contractor, but obviously at high cost. This area is governed by the duty of care under the **Environmental Protection Act 1990**.

**Q131 I am aware that chlorine-based chemical sanitisers affect aluminium and anodised surfaces, including shelving and meat slicers. How can I ensure adequate sanitisation of such equipment?**

A This is certainly a problem and a drawback in the use of such sanitisers. Ice-cream scoops are similarly affected, often causing pitting, which may harbour bacteria. In such circumstances it is better to use quaternary ammonium compound sanitisers; whilst these are generally slow acting and have to be in contact with the surface for a 5–10 minute period to ensure sanitisation, they are the best option under the circumstances.

**Q132 What is the best method of ensuring the proper sanitisation of ice-cream scoops between use?**

A The ideal situation is that an ice-cream scoop is kept in warm running water between each use. It is possible to install devices which allow for this but this should only generally be considered where large quantities of ice cream are being served, eg specialist ice-cream retail operations. The next best method would be the use of quaternary ammonium compound sanitisers, which should be mixed with warm water in a small upright container. The ice-cream scoop can be left in this solution between use. If extensive use is made then it would be necessary to change the solution frequently.

**Q133 Can my polypropylene cutting boards be put through the dishwasher before routine cleaning?**

A This is certainly the best method of cleaning them. Many caterers do this as a matter of routine; however, thin boards may be prone to warp over a period of time given the high temperature of the rinse water. Thick boards certainly are not prone to the same physical damage and can be cleaned in this way. Some of the larger boards may obstruct the washing arms of the dishwasher, therefore not allowing the dishwasher to achieve the desired results.

**Q134 How should I store my cutting boards?**

A Cutting boards should be stored so that they can be protected against risk of contamination, eg not under tabling where food debris may spill onto them, and certainly off the floor where they may easily become contaminated. The best method is by using a vertical rack which separates the boards and ensures that they will always air dry after cleaning. This will prevent mould and bacterial growth which is a common occurrence when they are stored wet and flat together. Racks should be stainless steel and can be purchased through many catering suppliers.

**Q135 What does the term "clean as you go" mean and how can it best be achieved?**

A "Clean as you go" is simply the process of cleaning up after you complete a particular task within the food preparation area, not leaving all cleaning until the end of the day. By doing a little cleaning often, it prevents the likelihood of standards dropping over time. It can best be achieved through good staff training and supervision and the use of written cleaning schedules.

**Q136 Is there any benefit from segregation of waste in my business? It seems that the cost of general waste disposal is increasing all the time.**

A If you are a business that sells packaged goods to the final consumer you may need to register with the Environment Agency or Scottish Environmental Protection Agency as required by the **Producer Responsibility Obligations (Waste Packaging) Regulations 1997**. You will need to register if your business has a turnover of over £5 million per year (£1 million from 1 January 2000) and produces more than 50 tonnes of packaging waste per year. You will then need to recover and recycle specific tonnages of packaging waste. Segregation of your waste will allow easier calculation of the amount of packaging waste you use and make recycling easier. Segregation may also allow you to separate items for different means of disposal. For example, you may wish to separate food waste from non-putrescible waste (such as plastic, wrapping — anything that won't decompose) in order to ensure that bins do not overflow with rubbish that will attract pests.

**Q137 How can chemical contamination be prevented if chemicals are put onto food surfaces to kill bacteria?**

A This is the perennial dilemma of achieving good disinfection without chemically contaminating food. Most proprietary sanitisers will clean and disinfect in one operation and can be left in place on the food contact surface without causing contamination. They are termed “food safe” but you should always read the label and ensure the recommended concentration is used.

# BARS AND CELLARS

**Q138 To what standard should I maintain my cellars structurally, as I understand they are classed as food rooms under the law?**

A This has been the subject of much debate amongst enforcement officers and the trade. Guidance to enforcement officers from the Local Authorities Co-ordinating Body on Trading Standards (LACOTS) has suggested that cellars are low-risk areas, only requiring minimal upkeep and potential for cleaning.

Cellar ceilings and walls should be in a good state of repair and free from mould growth, leaks and water penetration and obvious damage and holes. Painting with white, thick, emulsion paint on an annual or perhaps bi-annual basis will maintain the surface and improve appearance. This can be done over any brickwork, blockwork, etc and there is no real need for plastering. The floor can be bare concrete and provided it is in good condition without obvious holes and cracks there should be little comment from inspectors. Adequate drainage is necessary to ensure wet washing can easily be undertaken each day under stillages and in corners and edges. Lighting and good ventilation together with air cooling are obviously essential for safety and product quality.

**Q139 What are the requirements for bottle stores?**

A There is no legal requirement with respect to empty bottle stores as these in no way could be classed as food rooms. However, under health and safety law, in particular the **Workplace (Health, Safety and Welfare) Regulations 1992**, repair of the floor, walls and ceilings should be adequate, with good lighting and ventilation also required in these areas. Such circumstances demonstrate a tidy business, maintaining the asset and providing for a pleasant working environment for staff.

**Q140 What facilities with respect to sinks, etc should be provided in my beer store?**

A LACOTS advice to enforcement officers suggests that only a sink with access to cold water is necessary. Wash-hand basins with all their associated facilities are not really necessary as all "foods" handled within the beer store are low risk and enclosed in barrels. It is also useful to have a hose permanently attached to the tap for floor washing but this is not a legal requirement.

**Q141 How often should I clean my beer lines?**

A This depends on usage; however, yeast and other spoilage organism build up can occur within a few days. Weekly cleaning should be a minimum. Care should be taken to flush through all beer-line cleaning fluid once the operation has been undertaken. Serious accidents have occurred when adequate attention to cleaning has not been taken.

**Q142 What washing facilities do I require in my bar area?**

A The staff side of the bar is classed as a food area because of the handling of open drinks and snacks. Therefore handwashing facilities are essential with soap and towel; these should be separate from any glass-washing facilities. A double drainer is usually required for glass-washing so that one can adequately wash and sanitise glasses in two processes. This could be undertaken in one process for small bars. However, a glass-washer would usually be available in addition to any sinks provided and cannot replace them as access to water is often needed. Water should not be drawn from the glass-washer because of the risk of contamination.

**Q143 Why is there a need for a wash-hand basin in a bar area when only low-risk food products are handled?**

A The main reasons are as follows:

- often dirty bottles are handled, causing hand contamination which needs to be removed
- there is a need to touch and cut fruit for drinks which may lead to contamination
- ice should be handled only with tongs, but the tongs sometimes come in contact with the glass leading to possible contamination
- the rims of glasses are handled, sometimes excessively, and they have to come in contact with the lips of the customers which may provide a risk of food-borne infections

- contact with chemicals during glass-washing or after other bar cleaning processes may lead to chemical contamination of glasses if handwashing facilities are not available.

**Q144 Are there any risks from open snacks such as crisps, nuts, pickled onions, gherkins, dips, etc on the bar?**

A There have been a number of studies undertaken which demonstrate that contamination of these products does occur with bacteria including Staphylococcus and Escherichia coli. Foreign material contamination by hairs, fingernails, etc can also occur. There is, however, little risk of food poisoning as such products are often either extremely salty or pickled. Only when mayonnaise and other high-risk dip products are used may there be some risk. It is important to ensure that such items are kept to a minimum in small bowls and regularly replenished from fresh supplies.

**Q145 What is the best method to dispense nuts at the bar to reduce contamination?**

A Dispensing machines are available that will provide protection from contamination. Alternatively, provide the very small foil packets (as found on airlines). Thin-necked jugs will prevent contamination, as people will not be able to handle the nuts easily. If this is impractical, ensure that the bowl is filled with the minimal amount and replenished regularly.

**Q146 What is the best type of hand-drying facility in bar areas?**

A Certainly in such circumstances air hand-dryers would be out of the question because of the noise. It is not advisable to use cloths as these can inadvertently be used for glassware and wiping down processes. The best method by far would be disposable paper towels from a dispenser situated under the bar surface area.

**Q147 What is the best method of glass storage within the bar area?**

A Glasses need to be adequately cleaned and dried before storage, otherwise bacteria, moulds and stains will be a problem. It is not illegal to dry and polish glasses with a clean dry cloth, but air drying after removal from a glass-washer is preferable. Air drying can be assisted by ensuring the glasses are washed in extremely hot water for the final rinse and then stored on open plastic mats which allow air to circulate under the rim of the glass. Glasses should never be stored directly onto formica or other surfaces. Bar staff should always check every glass for signs of stains before it is used.

**Q148 How should I store spirit measures to prevent contamination?**

A There is a risk of contamination, particularly from foreign matter and fruit flies; however, these risks are slight. Storage under a shelf at the back of the bar is adequate and obviously when the measures are not in use they should be stored inverted. Cleaning in a chlorine-based sanitiser in a weak solution is recommended; however, care should be taken not to taint drinks with residue. Only stainless steel measures should be treated in this way; others may be damaged by such solutions. Quaternary ammonium compounds are recommended as an alternative.

**Q149 Is there any risk from selling out-of-date bottled beverages? Am I in breach of any statute if I do so?**

A Beers, ciders and fruit juices are now all labelled with a "best before" date which should be adhered to. The life of such beverages is difficult to anticipate and will depend on storage temperature and conditions. A business that is well run would never exceed such dates as it would ensure stock rotation.

**Q150 Can I legally recover beers drawn through but not consumed? They appear to be slightly cloudy, particularly at the start and end of the barrel.**

A There is a risk of contamination from such residues depending on the circumstances. This may occur because of the container into which they are placed and also from the bar environment. It is not recommended that such products are re-used as this may lead to the contamination of the whole barrel. It is not, however, strictly illegal, providing that you can prove there is no risk of contamination. Most enforcement officers would tend not to agree with you, however. Certainly the beer residues in drip trays should never be re-used.

**Q151 Is there any risk from service of main meals over the bar as well as beverages?**

A The risks are only those that can normally be anticipated, including contamination from the environment and inadequate temperature control. Provided that food is served quickly and only passes through and over the counter, there is little risk. Adequate handwashing facilities should be maintained and food should not be left on the bar for long periods at ambient temperatures. Any sandwiches, pies, etc should be properly enclosed or wrapped and temperature control, hot or cold, should be maintained. There may be quality issues to be considered, including that of greasy marks to glassware, but such issues have long been resolved by separate areas for service, dedicated staff and good quality dishwashers. There should be no real conflict of interest.

**Q152 What may be classed as reasonable protective clothing for use in a bar area?**

A Staff do not have to wear hats or any particular overalls since such service is a low-risk operation. It is recommended, however, that an apron of some form be used as this will protect any food and beverages from contamination from outdoor clothing and also help to create a positive corporate image for the company. It would have a secondary role in protecting workers' clothes from spillages which can create a negative image in the minds of customers.

**Q153 What are the rules on smoking in bar areas?**

A Smoking is expressly forbidden under the **Food Safety (General Food Hygiene) Regulations 1995** and no bar or waiting staff are allowed to smoke whilst handling food. There is a risk of contamination and an enforcement officer may prosecute if staff were seen smoking in or around the bar area. Wash-up areas, cellars, bottle stores and other associated areas would also be out of bounds for smoking purposes.

# FOOD HYGIENE TRAINING

**Q154 Is there a legal requirement to carry out food hygiene training?**

A The **Food Safety (General Food Hygiene) Regulations 1995** state that supervision, instruction and/or training "commensurate with work activity" shall be undertaken.

**Q155 What recognised training courses are available in food hygiene and who carries them out?**

A There are four main bodies which certify training in the UK.

- The Chartered Institute of Environmental Health (CIEH), tel: 020 7928 6006.
- The Royal Environmental Health Institute of Scotland, tel: 0131-225 5444.
- The Royal Society of Health, tel: 020 7630 0121.
- The Royal Institute of Public Health and Hygiene, tel: 020 7580 2731.

All the above organisations certify training to three levels.

- Level 1: Basic or primary — generally a six hour course for all food handlers. "Options", a modular basic course from the CIEH, is also available.
- Level 2: Intermediate — generally a three-day course for supervisors.
- Hazard analysis or HACCP training course — usually 10 hours or more, for managers.
- Level 3: Advanced or diploma level — usually a five-day (40 hour) course for managers.

These courses are run by accredited centres which include consultants, local authorities, colleges, or possibly in-house within companies depending upon the level of expertise available. It is possible to train a person within the organisation to advanced or diploma level and if they acquire suitable experience in trainer skills they would be allowed to register as a centre and teach their own staff at primary level. General intermediate and advanced level courses are not carried out in-house, however, because a percentage of the teaching has to be undertaken by a qualified environmental health officer or other suitably accredited person.

**Q156 To what level should I train my staff in food hygiene?**

A This is specified in the *Industry Guide to Good Catering Practice* from the CIEH, and depends upon a number of criteria.

- The type of work undertaken by the staff member — it is fair to assume that persons handling low-risk foods or foods that are not "open" do not have to have the same level of training as, for example, chefs or those engaged in handling high-risk foods. Bar staff and waiting staff may also only require rudimentary food hygiene training.
- The nature of the business — where the company uses much technology, eg cook-chill, sous vide, vacuum-packing, preparation of large quantities of cooked meats, sausages, etc, then a high degree of training is needed for all workers involved with these processes.
- The size of the business — in multi-site operations where food may be transferred within the company, there are inherent risks for which those involved would need particular training.
- Status of individuals within the company — managers and supervisors are likely to want a higher level of training than basic grade food handlers so that adequate supervision can be carried out.
- Particular jobs — a training manager, for example, would need to acquire a higher level of knowledge in order to train others. A manager responsible for carrying out audits or dealing with environmental health officers would also need a higher level of knowledge.

**Q157 What subjects should be covered on a basic food safety course undertaken "in-house" within a catering business?**

A The following would be appropriate:

- basic introduction — the need for good food hygiene standards
- basic bacteriology including three main bacteria, ie Salmonella, Clostridium perfringens and Staphylococcus aureus
- pest identification, control and prevention
- personal hygiene

- cleaning theory and practice
- design
- delivery, storage and preparation of foods
- relevant legislation, ie the requirements of the **Food Safety Act 1990** and **Food Safety (General Food Hygiene) Regulations 1995**.

It may be possible to undertake such a course in about six hours, split over a number of days or weeks, or the CIEH "Options" course may be used. However, some areas could be removed for shorter sessions providing the main points of personal hygiene, knowledge of temperature control and cross-contamination and basic bacteriology are well covered.

**Q158 If food handlers have obtained their basic food hygiene certificate, how frequently should they receive refresher training?**

A This depends very much on the quality of training given at basic level, as retention is directly proportional to the teaching methods used and the quality of the presenter. The catering manager should carry out regular audits of the premises having trained the staff (or had the staff trained) and if the practices have not improved one must question whether the training has been effective.

With so many legal changes and "new" bacteria gaining prominence over the last few years, there is a need now to update all food hygiene training. It would not be too much to consider annual refresher training for all those carrying out the basic food hygiene course, perhaps for an hour or two each year, and consider the retake of the course every three to four years, depending on the assessment of training needs already suggested.

Much depends on other measures being undertaken by the organisation. If regular audits are being undertaken and points brought to the attention of managers and staff, then obviously it is more likely that hygiene measures are being put into practice and in the process are being learnt by the staff. If there is a good food hygiene framework in the form of a company food safety policy with regular training on its requirements, then this could be considered to be part of the food hygiene refresher. It would certainly seen by the staff as a good reason for training rather than just training for training's sake.

**Q159 I have a busy catering organisation and find it extremely difficult to release staff and managers for any training. What are my options?**

A It is essential to provide training in all aspects of business, including customer care, sales, health and safety and food safety. Without these the business will not thrive in today's environment. There are a number of management courses available.

- Advanced and intermediate courses undertaken on a non-intensive basis perhaps for one day or half a day each week for 6–12 weeks for an advanced course, 3–6 weeks for an intermediate.
- Open learning for basic level courses, particularly with colleges.
- Future options — CD-ROM (compact disc — read only memory) products are likely to become available which can be used in conjunction with the company's display screen equipment and which a manager or staff member can use to undertake an interactive course at their own pace.

**Note:** It is important to plan training adequately with regard to shift patterns, leave periods and available time. Certainly many mistakes are made by training managers imposing strict training regimes on staff in rest periods or perhaps out of hours when they may not wish to undertake such intensive training activities. It may be a better option to plan production and perhaps alter it a few mornings a week when staff and managers are more likely to be amenable to training sessions.

**Q160 How do food hygiene qualifications tie into National Vocational Qualifications (NVQs)?**

A NVQs are principally "vocational" qualifications, eg catering, housekeeping, etc and whilst food hygiene plays a part and is written into the standards, food hygiene is not a vocation that stands on its own. There is a move, however, to grade these courses but a lead body has not yet been agreed and therefore little has been done to assess the courses.

**Q161 What is the best advice to help me pass my Advanced Food Hygiene exams? I have not done an exam for 20 years!**

A You're fortunate, as I write the CIEH Advanced Food Hygiene Questions, and I would say in recent years I have had people like yourself in mind. You should find the exam questions more practical and the structure of the questions more easily understood, using real life situations. My advice would be to do the following.

- Ensure you do well in your assignments: high marks in these makes it easier in the exam. Good research for the assignment is important and remember any work submitted must be your own.
- Do structured revision in line with the syllabus. You never know what's on the exam paper but you can guarantee the questions will be selected from across the syllabus.
- Read your notes, any course book provided and this Question and Answers book. You will find the Food Sources, Manufacturing and Food Preservation sections particularly useful as a quick revision guide.
- Read the exam question — so many candidates do not do this and often give totally irrelevant answers.
- Timing is important. You must time each question and finish the paper.
- Pick the best questions for you.
- Go back over the paper at the end — the later questions will often jog your memory for the earlier ones.
- Show your breadth of knowledge and give examples.
- If you follow these simple rules combined with some preparation after the course your chances of success are much higher.

**Q162 I am a manager in a catering industry who has only ever done a Basic Food Hygiene course. I have been asked by my boss to do an Advanced Food Hygiene course but confess to being worried about stepping up to that level without doing an Intermediate level first. What are my options?**

A If you have a lot of experience in the industry and are involved to some extent in food hygiene management as part of your job then there is no reason why you should not do your Advanced course without doing the Intermediate level. If you are worried about the challenge of the exam having not sat one for some years, see Q161 above. It may, however, be advisable to pass the Intermediate course first.

# FOOD POISONING AND FOOD COMPLAINTS

**Q163 Is the increase in reported cases of food poisoning a reflection of greater public awareness or an indication of generally lower standards in catering?**

A The increase in food poisoning is due in the main to the following.

- Intensive farming due to increasing demand for foods such as poultry, eggs, pre-packed meats, etc.
- Use of technology in the home and in catering including microwaves, freezers, chillers — abuses of such equipment are common and therefore food poisoning can result.
- Increasing amount of ready-prepared meals.
- Lack of general hygiene awareness with respect to foods such as chicken and raw eggs; even now some caterers still make egg mayonnaise without suitable regard for temperature control.
- A change in the foods consumed over the last 20–30 years — for example an increase in consumption of fast foods and ethnic foods like Chinese, Indian, kebabs, etc; there are some specialist organisms (eg Bacillus cereus) which affect these particular foods.
- An increase in exotic holidays and travel — infections are often imported, eg Typhoid, Dysentry, Campylobacter, Salmonella food poisoning.

**Q164 I have had, on occasions, complaints from customers that they have eaten food which has caused them food poisoning. How can I ascertain whether they are justified and what is the best means by which to deal with such complaints?**

A All businesses involving catering will, from time to time, have allegations made against them from customers. Often there is another underlying problem which may be of a hygiene or service-related nature. Such complaints are likely to be received in the following ways.

- From the customer staying overnight — in the morning prior to payment of the bill.
- By telephone, perhaps days after the meal.
- By letter which could be up to several weeks after the meal.
- Via the local authority environmental health officer.

**DEALING WITH FOOD POISONING COMPLAINTS**

It should be remembered that all food poisoning complaints are "allegations" until they are proved otherwise. Depending on how the complaint is received, it is important to gain the following information if possible at the first point of contact with the customer:

- name, address and telephone number of the affected person(s)
- date and time the meal was consumed
- number of persons in party and number affected
- details of symptoms, eg diarrhoea, vomiting, stomach pains, fever, etc
- food consumed — obtain a menu and relate the complaint to what is on that menu to remind the customer
- date and time that the symptoms commenced after the food was consumed
- duration of the illness
- whether the customer has been to the doctor.

It is important that all staff are prepared to receive this information and they must gain it in a friendly "chatty" way rather than reading out questions from a pre-prepared sheet. There is usually only one opportunity to gain such information. Other telephone calls to the customer may give the impression that you are rather too concerned and may imply "the compensation cheque is on the way". From these details,, it may be possible to refute food poisoning altogether.

For example, the incubation period indicated may be considered to be too short for the symptoms given or the types of foods which allegedly caused the illness may not normally be responsible for causing that type of food poisoning. In some cases, however, a further investigation will need to be made.

**THE INVESTIGATION**

A close study of the menu with the chef is necessary to identify possible shortcomings in preparation methods. It could be assumed that if the food was prepared in a safe way, with necessary regard for food hygiene, then it should not have caused food poisoning. Details of suppliers, dates when food was supplied, etc should also be investigated. The total number of meals served of a similar nature should be taken into account and if no other complaints have been received from consumers of the same dish this will be an advantage. An inspection of the kitchen with regard to temperature control and cross-contamination risks is necessary. The state of health of the chef a week or perhaps two weeks prior to the alleged incident together with any sore throats, cuts, boils and sores on hands, etc must also be thoroughly investigated.

**FOOD SAMPLES**

It would be an advantage if samples had been kept from a function or prepared food items, as these could be tested by a laboratory to ascertain if any pathogenic (food poisoning) bacteria are present. The role of independent consultants in carrying out this investigation and liaising with the customer cannot be overemphasised. Impartiality can be of great assistance to caterers in establishing their innocence.

**IMMEDIATE ACTION**

Having received the initial complaint, it would be advantageous to write to the customer and say that the matter is being fully investigated and they will be contacted again once this investigation has been completed. This can have the effect of allying fears that the incident is not being taken seriously. Usually the customer will not contact the establishment or other agencies with respect to the matter until the manager makes contact with them.

| FINAL ACTION |
| --- |
| Once an investigation has been completed, it is important to let the customer know of the findings, and these should be given in broad terms only. They should not be given any details as it is always possible that they may misinterpret any minor problem found as the cause of their particular incident, which may not have been the case. Should the unfortunate situation occur that suspicious circumstances do emerge from the investigation, then it would be better to be fair and honest and inform the local authority enforcement officer who should be reasonable providing satisfactory due diligence systems are in place. |

**Q165 What should I do if I believe food poisoning complaints are justified?**

A It is always extremely difficult to find an easy answer to this problem, particularly when you may be at fault. The best policy is honesty and you should immediately contact an environmental health consultant or your local authority environmental health department for advice. Be aware that if they find unsatisfactory conditions, they may consider prosecution and they will wish to see all your records and any food hygiene measures which you are undertaking.

It would be helpful to them to have the following documents available:

- the company's overall policy with respect to food hygiene
- details of any temperature monitoring or other records including training, etc that may be available
- any details that are available with regard to the menu, its preparation and handling of each food
- details of suppliers, delivery dates, quantities, etc
- details of any other related complaints received.

This policy of honesty is likely to be well received by the enforcement officers. To hide the problem is likely to result in a harder line being taken. It may be deemed a criminal offence not to report any food samples which are available.

**Q166 Is it useful to take food samples of foods that I prepare in case complaints of food poisoning are received?**

A The difficulty is that food samples are not always representative of foods served. For example, if one was catering for a large banquet where several joints of beef were prepared, which beef joints should be sampled — all of them, or just one? Nevertheless, there is some value in saving high-risk foods, particularly when carrying out extensive function work. Certainly most reputable companies would carry out this practice as a routine and the following is offered as guidance.

- Only keep samples for major functions, eg over 50 persons.
- Take only high-risk food samples, eg meats, gravies, fish, products made from egg, rice, etc. At least 100g of each food should be taken and they should be placed in clean, preferably sterile, containers or plastic bags and then frozen or kept in a refrigerator.
- Keep samples for about one week (they do build up incredibly quickly if there is a large amount of function work).
- Have ready the telephone number of a laboratory that can carry out such food sampling work.

**Q167 What is the benefit of submitting food samples for analysis? What bacteria should I have the food analysed for?**

A Certainly there is great advantage in occasionally submitting for analysis foods which have been prepared at your catering business. This can demonstrate good due diligence in that you are indicating that you wish to ensure good food handling standards. The process can identify shortcomings in cleaning or cross-contamination and temperature control.

A general screen should be requested together with analysis of a number of particular bacteria, depending on the type of food. A general screen is likely to cost around £25 and will involve the following.

- TVC (total viable count) — this is the total number of organisms found, whether pathogenic or spoilage.
- Escherichia coli — this is principally a human gut bacteria but can be found in other animals
- Other coliforms — these indicate contamination levels within the kitchen.

**Q168 When should I inform the EHO that my organisation may have caused a food poisoning incident?**

A At the earliest opportunity when the cases reach six or more. The temptation is that if you don't mention the subject you won't be found out. This is highly unlikely when large numbers are affected. Complaints from people who attended the function or the results of faecal samples will notify the environmental health officer anyway. The EHO may be more lenient with you if you show yourself to be proactive and co-operative. Early investigation of the problem will also prevent any further spread of the illness.

**Q169 What is the best way of dealing with a customer who finds a foreign object in their food?**

A Initially you should attempt to gain possession of the object. This should be done politely on the basis that you will investigate the source of the object. If the customer is unwilling to give you the object you must respect this but request that you have sight of it. You must then try to identify the source of the object. If the object's source is your own premises, and the customer takes their complaint to the EHO, you may be prosecuted if you are unable to prove "due diligence". If the source is one of your suppliers, you should contact them to see what precautions they take to prevent such occurrences (manufacturing records such as metal-detector checks will help you with this). If you are not happy with the response you should consider changing supplier.

**Q170 Is it not best to offer a small token in compensation at the table in the case of food complaints?**

A By offering a token gesture you may be unwittingly admitting liability for the complaint. It is best to carry out a full investigation prior to making any offers. If the customer merely wishes to have their money back then this would be acceptable.

| THE SPECIFIC BACTERIA |
|---|
| • Salmonella — usually screened to ensure chicken and egg products are uncontaminated. Any presence would be unsatisfactory<br>• Clostridium perfringens — usually undertaken for meat products and can demonstrate the quality of mince and other such foods.<br>• Staphylococcus aureus — usually indicates deficient standards of food handling as it is a normal organism found on the skin and in the mouth or throat of humans.<br>• Bacillus cereus — usually undertaken for rice, pasta and other wheat-based and cereal-based products.<br>• Vibrio parahaemolyticus — undertaken for prawns and other seafoods; usually indicates poor quality, depending on origin. |

**Q171 What is the true incidence of food poisoning within the UK?**

A A recent Department of Health study estimates that 9.4 million cases of "Intestinal Infectious Disease" occur in England each year and from this figure it is possible to predict cases for Scotland, Wales and Northern Ireland. This is an estimate and it is for all intestinal illness including viral gastroenteritis which is not always caused by food. The main organisms involved are Campylobacter (4.2%) and salmonella (1.1%) but these are only the identified cases. It is likely that millions of affected people suffer in silence without going to their doctor.

**Q172 What is the financial cost of food poisoning in the UK?**

A From a recent Department of Health study the estimate for England was around £743 million per year.

# HAZARD ANALYSIS AND ASSURED SAFE CATERING

**Q173 I have heard much about HACCP and hazard analysis. What does this mean and is it of any value to my catering business?**

A HACCP stands for "Hazard Analysis and Critical Control Points". It was developed in the USA for processing of zero-defect food for space flights. The concept has certainly been used in food manufacture for many years and does have a place within the catering environment. The **Food Safety (General Food Hygiene) Regulations 1995** require all caterers to carry out some form of hazard analysis and identification of critical controls. The basic steps are as follows.

- Evaluation of hazards — an inspection of the catering unit should be undertaken to establish what are the main hazards which may cause physical, chemical or biological risk to food. An assessment of the risk should be undertaken and these matters dealt with by the following means:
  - elimination
  - substitution
  - containment
  - safe systems of work, or
  - control of personnel, including personal protective equipment.
- Development and implementation of controls — it is necessary to identify critical control points which affect food safety and develop systems by which these can be measured regularly to provide documentary evidence that controls are in place. A critical control point is that which, if not undertaken, will adversely affect the food. It may include the following parameters:
  - time
  - temperature
  - density
  - weight
  - volume
  - packaging.

- Evaluation of controls — this is the periodic evaluation to check that the systems remain in operation. It may involve the occasional checking of one particular food through the system or an audit of the whole system to ensure it is working. This has a central place within catering and should be undertaken within all catering establishments.

**Q174 What is the difference between HACCP and hazard analysis?**

A Hazard Analysis and Critical Control Points (HACCP) is a specific type of hazard analysis. It was first used in the 1970s as part of NASA's space programme. Prior to this, the emphasis had been put on dealing with the final product (end-product testing). HACCP is product specific and requires in-depth microbiological and scientific knowledge. It can also take up a large amount of time and investment. This is not always practical for smaller businesses with a variety of products. As a result, other hazard analysis (the overall term) concepts have been developed (such as assured safe catering).

**Q175 What do I need to know about hazard analysis?**

A Hazard analysis is a management system designed to maintain food safety. Hazard analysis identifies "critical control points" in the production steps of food. By controlling these critical points, food safety is achieved. A critical control point is when a process or action reduces the risk posed by a food hazard to an acceptable level. For instance, cooking destroys Salmonella bacteria and is therefore a critical control point. This process can be carried out for all steps in food production, thus ensuring food safety. Hazard analysis of some description is a legal obligation under the **Food Safety (General Food Hygiene) Regulations 1995**.

**Q176 What training should I undertake to carry out my own hazard analysis?**

A You should have sufficient technical expertise to carry out a hazard analysis. If you are the manager of a large organisation, you will probably have much of the expertise required already. However, in a smaller business where you may be responsible for all aspects of the hazard analysis, Intermediate or Advanced Food Hygiene should be seen as a starting point. These courses will provide you with the technical knowledge required. Courses are now available in hazard analysis which will teach you how to carry out the actual assessment.

**Q177 What should my staff know about hazard analysis?**

A Your staff should be involved in the hazard analysis process from the outset. Your staff will have an in-depth knowledge of the processes involved and will be able to advise you of the current situation and the likely hazards. As part of your hazard analysis you should set up a team, pulling together all the key staff. This will ensure that not only will the hazard analysis be accurate, it will also be used by the staff.

**Q178 How can "critical control points" be easily identified?**

A A critical control point (CCP) is defined as a step in the food production process that will eliminate or reduce a hazard to an acceptable level. Using the technical knowledge you have gained through your training, you will be able to identify the hazards associated with your operation. Once you have identified the hazards, you must decide what controls are in place (eg refrigeration, cooking, etc). If a control is essential to food safety then it is classified as a CCP (eg cooking). If a control is not essential then it is not a CCP (eg refrigeration of raw meat, although good practice, is not a CCP because the meat will be cooked).

**Q179 How can my catering business cost-effectively operate a hazard analysis (HACCP) system as required by the regulations?**

A It is extremely difficult to implement traditional HACCP systems within catering operations. The difficulty lies in the fact that this system was developed for food manufacturing and is more appropriately implemented on production lines. Catering businesses do not have clear food flows, particularly those which are of a hotel or restaurant nature. The best hope would be to attempt the Department of Health assured safe catering concept. This deals with the food flow more globally throughout the whole of the unit and involves the identification of critical points (critical control points), which if not undertaken correctly to the required standard may run the risk of causing food poisoning.

With such a new field of expertise needed it may be advantageous to employ a good consultant.

**Q180 What is a practical way of complying with the legal requirements for hazard analysis?**

A The **Food Safety (General Food Hygiene) Regulations 1995** require that "a proprietor of a food business shall identify any step in the activities of the food business which is critical to ensuring food safety and ensure that adequate safety procedures are identified, implemented, maintained and reviewed." As you can see, it does not require a full-blown HACCP — indeed it does not even need to be documented. However, if you don't write the procedures down it may be difficult to show the EHO that you have carried them out. As a minimum you should draw a simple flow diagram for your business, showing the different steps in food preparation (eg delivery, storage, etc) and identify the hazards and control measures for each step. Records of checks carried out, such as temperature records and cleaning schedules, prove that you are monitoring the situation. Once you've done all this you should review the situation regularly or whenever there is a major change to the system.

**Q181 Is the concept of "assured safe catering" of use to my catering business?**

A Absolutely. For the majority of catering businesses, assured safe catering (ASC) is of more relevance than the traditional HACCP. HACCP is appropriate for manufacturing industries where there tend to be high volumes of a few products. As such, an HACCP can be carried out for all products. In a catering business this would not be practical due to the variety of products on offer. ASC assumes that certain steps are repeated whatever the food and general controls put in place (such as refrigerating all high-risk foods).

**Q182 What will the EHO do if I have not done a hazard analysis for my business?**

A Guidance on how EHOs enforce the law initially gave a run-in period of two years for businesses to get to grips with hazard analysis. This period ended on 15 September 1997. If standards of hygiene within your organisation are good it is likely that the EHO will take an informal approach. However, should standards be poor or your business causes a food poisoning outbreak, then you will almost certainly have formal action taken. This may take the form of an improvement notice or even prosecution.

**Q183 What are the key stages in carrying out Hazard Analysis?**

A There are seven key stages:

- Identification and analysis of food hazards.
- Identification of critical points.
- Deciding on controls and limits at critical points.
- Developing documentation for control monitoring.
- Deciding on corrective actions.
- Carrying out monitoring.
- Designing a review procedure.

**Q184 How can hazard analysis in my business be more clearly understood by my staff?**

A There are a number of practical measures you can take. The marking of places which are critical points is a good first measure together with making particular staff responsible for the monitoring of the point. This might mean they have to regularly monitor the food at that point and keep a record of it. The use of flow charts and pictorial explanations of what to do at each stage is a good idea.

**Q185 What, in a few words, is the simplest form of hazard analysis?**

A Whilst there are seven key stages of hazard analysis (see Q183 ) the monitoring of the control measures at critical points is the key issue that needs to be addressed.

**Q186 When monitoring a critical point in my catering operation, what should be recorded?**

A Such monitoring logs should cover all the essential factors affecting any particular point which might include:

- What controls are being monitored — cooking/cooling times, weight of product, date code, temperature, etc.
- Type of product.
- Frequency of monitoring.

- Period over which the point is being monitored.
- Who carries out the monitoring.
- Who checks to confirm recording is properly being carried out — is the probe calibrated for example.
- Any control targets to be achieved e.g. food to be delivered at 1°– 4° C but acceptable up to 8° C.

**Q187 When should I review my hazard analysis?**

A Without a review procedure all your efforts at hazard analysis will become redundant. There are key times when reviews should take place and these include the following.

- When new dishes/items are introduced onto the menus.
- If new equipment is introduced which modifies the food process e.g. blast chillers, convection ovens, etc.
- If purchasing specifications or arrangements change, e.g. if food is bought ready-prepared and frozen or you wish to now prepare your own desserts.
- If you receive food complaints which could lead you to redefine how you prepare food items.
- Upon advice from a visit by your EHO.
- When any sampling programme indicates that the food has unsatisfactory bacterial or chemical results, or there is evidence of physical contamination.

**Q188 Do I legally have to have a written record of my hazard analysis?**

A There is no legal requirement at present under the regulations to write down your hazard analysis but the Government is considering changing this in the future. The problem you have if you don't write it down is explaining it all to the EHO when they make a food safety inspection!

**Q189 What are my options if I cannot find the time to carry out hazard analysis myself within my operations?**

A Several options are possible which include those listed below.

- Engage a food safety consultant to do the work for you and ensure the system they develop is properly implemented and updated/reviewed.

- Send one of your key staff on a training course such as the CIEH Hazard Analysis Course, obtainable locally through one of the CIEH training centres (Tel: 020 7928 6006). Your staff member could then do the hazard analysis as part of his or her routine duties.
- Purchase one of the published products "Simply Safe" or "Assured", again obtainable through the CIEH. The manual can then be used as a guide to carry out the hazard analysis.
- Use some of the Croner's records in *Croner's Catering Records & Procedures* manual as the basis for monitoring of critical points.
- Consider the new ***Hamster*** © system from HMS Ltd (Hazard Analysis Monitoring System To Ensure Recording). Tel: 01225 858412.

**Q190 When might an EHO seize food and what are my rights in this respect?**

A Under the **Food Safety Act 1990** any "authorised officer" which usually include EHOs (see Q191) may seize or take possession of food that they consider is either unfit for human consumption or fails to meet food safety requirements. Essentially they have to take it before a magistrate who may then condemn the food to be destroyed. Authorised officers do not have the right to condemn food. You have the right to object to condemnation and are allowed before the magistrate to argue your case.

**Q191 Is it only EHOs who carry out food inspections?**

A No. The **Food Safety Act 1990** makes it a duty of all local authorities to inspect the food outlets in their areas for time to time. The authority must appoint Authorised Officers who carry out the inspections. These persons are often qualified environmental health officers who have a wide remit including food safety, health and safety, housing and pollution matters. It is common though, for these Authorised Officers not to be a qualified EHO but to have specialist technical qualifications just in the food safety field. Such persons are known as Technical Assistants and they often work under the direction of the EHO at the authority. Trading standards officers may also carry out food inspections to determine quality/labelling issues.

**Q192 What records do I need to keep to ensure I have a complete "due diligence" defence?**

A The key records needed these days are those which monitor the critical points in your catering operation. They may include a list of authorised/nominated suppliers, delivery monitoring, storage, preparation matters including defrosting procedures and cleaning records for food contact surfaces, cold food preparation monitoring, cooking temperature monitoring, cooking procedures, reheating and service monitoring. It may also be useful to record training status, pest control treatment, dishwasher maintenance/service and building maintenance. This list depends on your business activities.

**Q193 What will be the functions of the new Food Standards Agency?**

A Essentially this has yet to be decided, however they will include:

- developing policies and advising the Government and public authorities on food safety
- providing advice, information and assistance on food standards to the public and other interested parties
- obtaining and keeping under review information about food safety and related issues by commissioning research
- carrying out observations on the safety or quality of food at any point in the food chain for strategy purposes
- setting of standards for enforcement and monitoring the performance of food law enforcement authorities.

**Q194 Where can good, simple guidance on food law be obtained?**

A The industry guide to Good Catering Practice is by far the most useful and cost effective guide on the law to which caterers must comply. It provides interpretation of the legal requirement, guidance and good compliance codes. What is even more useful is that not only caterers consult them — enforcement officers also will use them during their inspections. There are guides for most sectors: retailers, market stalls, bakers, etc. and they are available from the CIEH via Chadwick House Group. Tel: 020 7928 6006.

# FOOD SAFETY LAW

**Q195 In plain language, what laws affect me in the catering business and what do I have to do?**

A This is a vast question but can be answered simply as follows.

**FOOD SAFETY ACT 1990**

This is the main piece of legislation governing the trading of food in any premises and there are a number of offences as follows.

- The sale or possession of food which fails to meet with food safety requirements. This includes:
  - food that is injurious to health,, eg containing chemicals which may cause injury to a person
    - unfit food — food which is mouldy or causes food poisoning
      - food which is so contaminated so as not to be fit for human consumption in that state, eg tainted with substances or dust and dirt.
- The sale of food which is not of the nature, substance or quality the customer demanded:
  - nature — food which is not as that described,, eg horse meat provided instead of beef
    - substance — food which contains foreign material including glass, cardboard, other packaging, etc
      - quality — the substitution of a lower quality food,, eg a rump steak instead of a sirloin or fillet.
- Obstructing an enforcement officer whilst carrying out his or her duty.
- Failing to comply with a notice or court order requiring work to the premises or closure.
- Falsely describing food — perhaps on menus or through advertising.

The Act also deals with enforcement powers, giving authorised officers the power to inspect, seize food, detain food, serve notices requiring work to be done to the premises, or closure, etc. The Act only deals with the movement and sale of food; it does not deal with the standards of hygiene within the premises.

**FOOD SAFETY (GENERAL FOOD HYGIENE) REGULATIONS 1995**

These regulations detail the hygiene standards required of premises. They are as follows.

- Proprietors of food businesses must carry out some form of hazard analysis.
- Food handlers must receive instruction,, supervision or training commensurate with their work activity.
- Staff must report any illness likely to be transmitted through the food.

The following are the "Rules of Hygiene". These are also legal requirements.

- Food premises must be kept clean and in good repair. Layout, design and construction must allow good food hygiene practices.
- Clean water, hand-washing facilities, toilets, ventilation, lighting, drainage and changing facilities for staff must be provided.
- Requirements for rooms where foodstuffs are prepared, treated or processed: floors, walls, ceilings, windows, doors and surfaces must be constructed of appropriate materials and must not pose a risk to food safety. Cleaning facilities must also be provided.
- Requirements for moveable and temporary premises: as above but includes detail on vending machines and domestic premises.
- Transport must be kept clean and in good repair and allow adequate separation of foods to prevent contamination and effective temperature control
- Equipment must be kept clean and constructed of materials that will not pose a risk to food safety. Each piece must be installed to allow adequate cleaning of the surrounding area.
- Food waste must not be allowed to accumulate in food rooms. Suitable arrangements for storage and disposal must be made.
- Water supply must be potable and adequate. Ice must be made from potable water.
- Personal hygiene must be maintained at all times. No person suffering from a disease likely to be transmitted through food shall be permitted to work as a food handler.
- The proprietor must be satisfied that foodstuffs are not contaminated before accepting them. Storage must prevent deterioration and protect from contamination. Pests must be controlled and hazardous substances labelled and stored in separate containers.

**FOOD SAFETY (TEMPERATURE CONTROL) REGULATIONS 1995**

These regulations detail the requirements for temperature control in food premises. The main provisions are as follows.

- Chilled foods must be kept at 8°C or cooler if they would become unsafe at temperatures above this.
- Manufacturers can recommend higher storage temperatures provided that safety is verified.
- Cold food for service or display can be kept above 8°C for a maximum of 4 hours.
- Hot food must be kept above 63°C. An exemption of 2 hours is allowed for service and display.
- All food is required to be kept under temperature control if this is necessary to maintain its safety.
- Food must be cooled quickly after heating or preparation.

**Q196 What are the benefits of the Food Safety Act 1990?**

A The Government certainly had a hard time in the late 1980s with numerous food scares including:

- Salmonella in eggs
- adulteration of Austrian wine with antifreeze and its subsequent import into the UK in vast quantities
- contamination of baby foods with foreign matter by criminal activity
- apparently new bacteria — Listeria listeriosis or Listeria monocytogenes in pâté, soft cheeses and other foods — causing a number of miscarriages and deaths
- botulism in hazelnut purée causing around 20 cases in the UK.

These incidents highlighted the need to improve enforcement and consider the ways in which technology had not eliminated but perhaps promoted food poisoning and adulteration of food. Ministers were given additional powers to stop suspect food in transit and enforcement officers were given powers to immediately close premises which were providing an imminent risk to health. The Act provided a framework for many new regulations which govern the hygiene of food and also implied a requirement for food hygiene training.

Whilst only Listeria appears to have been reduced in numbers, all other food poisoning is still increasing. There is, however, a better awareness within industry of the need to achieve standards and over the next five years the concept of "due diligence" will have an increasing effect with a more positive result.

**Q197 There have been many changes in food safety legislation. When are we likely to see some stability in this field so that caterers can catch up with those laws which are obviously essential?**

A Initially, the Government brought in the **Food Safety Act 1990** which revised the Food Act 1984. This was as a result of the food scares of the late 1980s. The Act gave increased powers to enforcement officers and created some new offences. Since then the Government has been working on EU directives, converting them into UK regulations; the EU has now taken over as the driving force with regard to food safety legislation. This is so that the EU can unify its legislation in the immediate future to make trade within the EU much more controlled. The main regulations have been about particular foods, eg red meat, poultry, fish and shellfish, game, eggs, milk and meat products. The overall hygiene in catering manufacturers' and retail premises is being controlled by the **Food Safety (General Food Hygiene) Regulations 1995**, the last major piece in the jigsaw. These require catering premises to be in a satisfactory condition and also require management systems to be in place for the purposes of hazard analysis and compulsory staff training. The Regulations came into force in September 1995 and there may be some other detailed regulations on the way, particularly in the wake of the increase in E.coli 0157 outbursts.

**Q198 How can I be sure that there will not be further U-turns in Government policy, which have up until now caused much unnecessary expenditure in my catering business?**

A Certainly there have been U-turns, particularly with regard to temperature control, but legislation often responds to crisis (for example the increase in E.coli outbreaks in the UK).

**Q199 Is the concept of all EU countries operating under and within the same hygiene legislation and guidelines an achievable reality or merely a bureaucrat's pipedream which only the UK will sign and enforce?**

A There is a general aim within Europe to have a similar legal framework within each Member State, whether it be health and safety, food safety, company law, or any other matter. Certainly food safety and health and safety have recently received much effort on behalf of the EU and the legislation is now similar throughout the whole of Europe, having been forced along through directives which each Member State has had to implement into national law. The UK has a strong national framework and a long history of rules and regulations in this field. It has a clear enforcement policy and well-established enforcement agencies. Not all other countries have had such strict enforcement and therefore have not developed the same philosophy with respect to these new rules. The level of compliance with EU directives is, in some cases, much lower than those found in the UK.

The main aim is to provide a situation whereby an importer of food can feel comfortable and safe in the knowledge that food from another Member State is prepared to the same standards to that at home. Someone in the position of importing products would be well advised to carry out a food hygiene audit rather than accept the guarantees that such producers might offer.

**Q200 Is there a legal requirement to refrigerate eggs?**

A No, the law is "silent" on eggs, milk and raw meat. It does not state that these three foods require temperature control. However, it is good practice to ensure that they are all temperature-controlled as they are perishable and possibly subject to micro-biological multiplication.

**Q201 I have mice in certain parts of the premises. Will I be closed down by the EHO?**

A Mice and other pests, including cockroaches and flies, are not uncommon in many premises throughout the UK. It is when they are closely associated with food areas that environmental health officers become concerned. In order to close a premises down, ie serve a prohibition notice on the owner, the officer will have to prove that the premises pose a risk to health. Premises have to be verminous, there has to be evidence of contamination of food, gross contamination, poor cleanliness or gross disrepair before closure can be considered. There is a legal requirement to attempt to exclude pests from food areas and also control them if they are present. However, providing that they are not causing an obvious contamination risk and they are being controlled, the officer should understand this situation.

**Q202 Is it a legal requirement to use colour-coded chopping boards?**

A Certainly not. There are many ways to reduce cross-contamination between raw and cooked foods and this is essentially what is required by law. Colour-coding is only an aid to segregation and it does not detract from the need to ensure proper sanitisation of surfaces which come into contact with food.

**Q203 Are fly-killing machines a legal requirement within premises?**

A No. A number of studies have demonstrated that fly-killing machines are ineffective against many types of flying insects. They often work by pure chance — the insect eventually flies into them, probably after having alighted on most of the surfaces in the kitchen already. They work best in darker areas away from fluorescent lighting but can actually be a food safety hazard themselves if they are situated above worktops and food production equipment — when the insect hits the high-voltage electrical grid, its head lands in the tray and its legs and wings drift gracefully onto the food being prepared.

Whilst they have a place in pest control, they are of little value when considering pest prevention. There is a school of thought that such machines, like all technology, give an air of responsible activity to enforcement officers with regard to this subject.

**Q204 An environmental health officer recently visited my food business and gave me a Food Safety Act notice requiring work to be carried out. I have insufficient time to do exactly what he requires; what are my options?**

A Enforcement officers are empowered under the **Food Safety Act 1990** to serve a notice to require certain works to be done. These works are deemed necessary because there has been a failure to comply with food hygiene and other regulations, therefore by implication the offences have already been committed. The notice provides a time period by which the works should be carried out and the following options are possible.

- You may ask for an extension of time if the works are extensive. The officer should reasonably allow for an extension to occur.
- You may suggest to the officer that other works of a lesser nature can be carried out which nevertheless will comply with the legal requirements. This may be more cost-effective.
- You may appeal against the notice to a magistrates' court on the grounds that the works are not necessary, but you must do this before the expiry of the notice.

Certainly you must not ignore the notice as this is a legal document and may result in prosecution, not just for breaches of food hygiene legislation but also for failing to comply with the notice.

**Q205 Can I refuse entry to an enforcement officer at times when we are extremely busy and ask them to visit at another time when we are more able to manage and deal with the situation?**

A No. Authorised officers are allowed under the **Food Safety Act 1990** to make a visit at any reasonable time; the term "reasonable time" means when you are operating and trading. It is quite legitimate for the officer to visit at a busy time to assess the standards of food handling being undertaken. In fact, such visits are far more beneficial in terms of enforcement than seeing empty kitchens with the power switched off.

**Q206 I have received summonses for food hygiene offences which allegedly occurred some time ago with respect to my business. I do not remember when the initial visit was undertaken, but it would appear now that the officer means business. Can they still take a case after such a long time period and what should be my next course of action?**

A Very much like other criminal offences (eg motoring offences), you find out formally through the post that the matter is being considered for prosecution through a summons which may be issued up to a year after the alleged offence. The process of prosecution of an alleged offender goes through a number of stages and can therefore take a long time. The prosecuting authority are allowed in law to take a case within three years of its discovery or one year from its commission. While this may seem rather unfair in terms of evidence and witnesses, it is not unheard of for summonses to be received within a month or so of becoming what is termed "statute-barred". The following actions should be considered.

- It is important to engage a solicitor who can represent your case in court and who has experience of similar cases.
- It may be worthwhile negotiating with the enforcement officers or their solicitors' department with respect to the summonses in order to reduce the numbers to a bare minimum. It would be worthwhile getting expert advice from an environmental health consultant.
- You have the option of a "due diligence" defence in law, which if put forward may avoid prosecution altogether. ("Due diligence" is extremely difficult to prove.) Considerable efforts will have to be made to ensure that good records have been maintained.
- An adjournment should be asked for in the first instance in order to gather thoughts and consider options.

**Q207 I understand that Food Safety Act cases are triable both in the magistrates' and crown courts. What would be the better option?**

A There are advantages and disadvantages either way, as shown in the table below.

| | ADVANTAGES | DISADVANTAGES |
|---|---|---|
| **MAGISTRATES' COURT** | Maximum penalties are less; £5000 or £20,000 per offence depending on which section of the Act or regulation applies. Maximum term of six months' imprisonment. | The case may not be as closely analysed as it would be in a crown court. The decision rests with one or maybe a small group of laypersons who may not understand the full legal situation with regard to food safety. |
| | Magistrates are laypeople and are solely responsible for judgment of the case. They are amenable to discussion and debate. | |
| | The case is likely to be over more quickly. | |
| | The case is likely to be less costly. Expensive barristers, whilst an option in the magistrates' court, would be a requirement in a crown court. | |
| **CROWN COURT** | There is more chance of acquittal, even in serious situations, as the case has to be proved beyond all reasonable doubt. Juries will certainly have considerable debate where there is any doubt. | High cost of case. Severity of penalties — unlimited fine for certain offences and up to two years in prison for most offences. More media attention and bad publicity if failure occurs. |

**Q208 I run a number of catering businesses in different areas of the country. I have noticed that the requirements of enforcement officers in one area may differ from those of officers in other areas. How can these inconsistencies be eliminated?**

A Inconsistency of enforcement has been a major issue over the past few years, particularly with new powers under the **Food Safety Act 1990.** A number of measures are being implemented to assist in this situation. These include the following.

- Home authority status — the head office of a company situated within a local authority area can apply to that authority for home authority status. When this is undertaken, an officer of the council will deal with all matters of advice appertaining to that business. Local authorities in other areas will be informed of this and they may still make inspections. However, if a situation arises where there is any debate, this will be dealt with by the home authority.

- Industry guides — the **Food Safety (General Food Hygiene) Regulations 1995** require industry guides to be written up by the trade. These will be approved by the Department of Health and ensure reasonable standards which are tailored to each particular type of industry, eg retail, manufacturing, frozen foods, distribution, catering, etc. Not only will enforcement be undertaken with respect to these regulations but it will have to be considered in the light of industry guides. This will add some consistency.

**Q209 How often do environmental health officers visit food premises and how can I anticipate when I might get an inspection?**

A There is no set requirement for enforcement officers to visit premises. However, the **Food Safety Act 1990** provides the power for this to occur and Code of Practice No. 9, *Food Safety Inspections,* provides a risk assessment format which should be completed and from this the frequency of visits is determined.

Some of the essential features are rather subjective and depend on the conditions found during the particular risk assessment.

**Q210 Yesterday my EHO inspected my premises and wasn't very happy to find that some issues which he had written to me about in the past had not been attended to. I tried to tell him that I ordered the parts necessary to comply with his previous letter, but he wouldn't listen. He said he was going to serve a "minded to" notice on me. What does this mean?**

A A "minded to" notice basically means that your EHO is minded to serve an improvement notice. It does not require you to carry out any work (this is what an improvement notice is for). Essentially they were introduced to allow proprietors a chance to make a representation to the EHO as to why an improvement notice is not necessary. In real terms it shows that your EHO is serious about making you comply with his previous letter. Prior to the introduction of "minded to" notices, your EHO would probably have served the improvement notice by now.

In this situation you have a good chance of preventing the service of the improvement notice. What you need to do is write to your EHO or speak to his Chief EHO, saying that the works will be carried out as soon as the parts arrive, and give a timescale. Note that if it is decided to not serve the improvement notice but you fail to carry out the work as agreed, you may be prosecuted.

**Q211 For how long is it recommended that food safety monitoring records be kept?**

A Such records are all the forms and logs used to monitor the critical points in your organisation and include: delivery monitoring, storage temperatures and stock control, cleaning schedules, cooking and reheating monitoring and service temperatures. It is difficult to say when they might be required and therefore should be kept for a sufficient amount of time to prove that they are part of the ongoing programme for the unit. The following is a guide:

- records maintained on site and in use — one month
- records archived — two years.

These measures would be appropriate in most circumstances.

**Q212 How can the catering manager be sure that staff actually follow the guidelines, instructions and policies laid down, apart from requiring them to attend training sessions and to complete and sign the relevant documentation and control forms?**

A This question raises a number of fundamental issues which underpin good food handling standards.

- Quality of staff — it is vital that high-quality staff who can demonstrate good hygienic practices are selected in the first instance. They need to be diligent, knowledgeable and have considerable common sense if they are to handle food safely. Qualifications, experience and training are extremely important and the latter must be ongoing throughout their period of employment with the company. If staff feel "cared for and developed", they will usually do a much better job.
- Training — new staff should be properly inducted into the company and made aware of the company policies and procedures. Training should be extremely visual, as practical as possible and dynamic enough to grab the trainees' attention and engender interest in what can be a very difficult and complex subject.

- Instruction — once training has been concluded, the next step is to instruct on a one-to-one basis in the workplace. This can be in the form of hazard-spotting and correction of defects or demonstrating procedures
- Supervision — even with the best procedures, without adequate supervision, staff may carry out activities outside the requirements of the policy. This may be because they are under pressure of work, because there are insufficient staff or perhaps because they have not had quite enough training. Young persons are particularly easily sidetracked and may not necessarily have a methodical approach. It is important that guidance on a one-to-one basis is always available and this must be allowed for in costings for catering work.
- Company policy — this must be easy to read, easy to follow and based on sound good practice. All aims, objectives and standards must be achievable and any such policy must be "owned" by the persons having to work with it. Policies must not be imposed upon the people within organisations but developed by them; that way staff are more likely to work with the system rather than against it.

Implementing the above measures should bring peace of mind with regard to the catering operation. At the end of the day, one can only do one's best. In the context of law, if a manager has done all that is reasonable then staff could be held responsible for their own acts or omissions.

**Q213 If I have suspected contamination of food within my catering business, do I have to retain the food and pass it on to the enforcement officer and, if so, how should it be kept prior to return or disposal?**

A It is illegal to possess food which fails to comply with food safety requirements. Nevertheless, such food may emerge from time to time and obviously there is a need for it to be clearly labelled if it is to be retained and sent back to the suppliers. Ideally it should be kept under refrigeration if it is a perishable product so that it does not decay further, as the supplier may think that the unit is responsible for its decay. Separate refrigerators or separate space within the same refrigerator, clearly labelled as such, is obviously necessary and the food should be returned to the supplier without undue delay.

There is no need or requirement to inform enforcement officers of such food. It is only if it is found by an enforcement officer that it may cause a problem.

**Q214 If high ambient temperatures within kitchens are a food safety risk, why is the law not stricter with respect to controlling ambient temperatures?**

A The **Food Safety (General Food Hygiene) Regulations 1995** require "adequate" ventilation in food rooms and this is open to much debate. Certainly good ventilation is essential, particularly at points where steam and hot equipment is situated, and between 12 and 20 air changes per hour would be necessary to achieve a satisfactory working environment. The ambient external air (ie the temperature outside) can raise temperatures internally to unacceptably high levels, particularly in the warm summer months. In such circumstances air cooling may be necessary. It is extremely difficult to achieve a satisfactory environment under all circumstances.

**Q215 How long can I leave sandwiches out at ambient temperature before I have to dispose of them?**

A This depends on when the sandwiches were produced and how they are being served. Any filling will deteriorate quickly and the bread will become dry and stale within a very short period of time, particularly if it is hot and dry. In terms of the present law, fresh sandwiches can be sold within four hours of the production time without having to refrigerate them. This can be done safely and is an exemption from the **Food Hygiene (Temperature Control) Regulations 1990.** In practice, one should not go much beyond four hours as such products are often handled excessively during preparation, introducing many bacteria of both a pathogenic and spoilage nature. Quality will suffer depending on the time and temperature of service. Refrigeration at below 5°C will prolong the life to up to 48 hours if necessary. This is most useful in vending and retail situations.

**Q216 What major changes did the Food Safety (General Food Hygiene) Regulations 1995 bring about?**

A The major changes were:

- legal requirement for management system with respect to hazard analysis of the business and implementation of control measures
- relaxation of temperature controls to 8°C
- compulsory food hygiene training for food handlers (commensurate with their work activity)
- requirement for fly screens to be fitted to windows that open "where appropriate"
- requirement that fly screens are demountable for cleaning
- requirement for access to ventilation systems for cleaning together with any filters and also access to fans
- equipment should be placed so as not to cause cleaning difficulties to the surrounding area (this has massive implications for small premises).

There is, however, a concession within the regulations in that there does not seem to be any mention of a requirement for nailbrushes to be provided.

In short, there would seem to be much leeway with respect to the 1995 regulations in that the words "adequate" and "where appropriate" have been placed within the text. This may in some cases benefit the proprietor but certainly will provoke much debate between proprietors and enforcement officers. The regulations have considerable implications with respect to such matters as fly screening and positioning of equipment. Demountability of such screening and movability of such equipment, together with accessibility of ventilation systems, are clearly defined and will have major cost implications for industry. Enforcement officers now have specific regulations dealing with matters that had previously not been dealt with in any depth by earlier legislation.

Enforcement officers will have the same powers under the **Food Safety Act 1990** to serve notices requiring work to be done if they deem it necessary.

**Q217 What are the temperature control requirements for caterers under the Food Safety (Temperature Control) Regulations 1995?**

A The Regulations brought in one single temperature of 8°C instead of the split between 5°C and 8°C for certain foods under the earlier temperature control requirements. All foods which may be host to microbiological multiplication or production of toxins must be subject to temperature control with the following exceptions.

- If the food is being prepared, cooked or served.
- A four-hour (ie one period of up to four hours) exemption for service is allowable at ambient temperature. Food for service which is not sold or served may be served from the refrigerator subsequently. The four-hour rule allows for sweet trolleys, cheese boards and ambient service at buffets, providing suitable prevention of contamination has been provided.

Hot food must be served at above 63°C. However, hot service below 63°C is allowable for up to two hours. Some businesses, such as take-away premises, would find this a great advantage. It would appear that, having prepared food freshly, they may be able to serve it at ambient temperature allowing it to cool over that period. Detailed guidance on temperature control has been revised and is available within the *Industry Guide to Good Catering Practice* from the CIEH. Tel: 020 7928 6006.

**Q218 What are the main differences in temperature control regulation in Scotland?**

A Although Scotland is governed by the same legislation (the **Food Safety (Temperature Control) Regulations 1995**) as England and Wales, the actual regulations are different. There is no legal maximum temperature for chilled foods in Scotland (8°C in England and Wales); "cold foods" are required to be kept in a cool place or refrigerator. Whilst the hot-hold temperature is the same (63°C), there are additional requirements to reheat food to 82°C and to boil gelatin or hold it at a minimum temperature of 71°C for 30 minutes in Scotland. There are a number of defences allowed in the English system for holding food outside the required temperatures. These are not available in Scotland, although certain exemptions are made.

**Q219 Do the Food Safety (General Food Hygiene) Regulations 1995 require small businesses to have details of hazard analyses in writing in case the inspector calls?**

A The Government and legislators recognise the increasing burden on businesses, particularly small businesses involved with food.

Enforcement officers are to have a new code of practice and the draft of this document suggests that hazard analysis does not necessarily have to be in writing. It would be very difficult to prove, however, that this had been carried out and small business proprietors might well struggle with questions asked by enforcement officers on this particular subject. It would seem that even small businesses should get training and guidance, and there is a need to have some form of commercially available format which is simple to complete and can be available to show such inspectors. In other words, whilst there is no legal requirement to detail matters in writing, it would be in the best interests of all business proprietors to do so.

**Q220 The term "adequate" appears open to much debate when considering food hygiene regulations. How can we be sure that we interpret this correctly?**

A Some law is drafted in an imprecise way to allow proprietors some leeway when implementing and complying with it. The 1995 regulations replaced the term "suitable and sufficient" with the words "adequate" and "where appropriate". Essentially these terms all mean the same thing. They do not directly commit the caterer to any particular standard and allow for interpretation by both the caterer and the enforcement officer.

Sadly, it is often for the courts to decide what the terms "suitable and sufficient", "where appropriate" or "adequate" actually mean and there has been much case law on matters such as the provision of suitable and sufficient wash-hand facilities. The higher the court making the decision, the more likely it is that the definition will influence future cases and therefore influence interpretation within industry. In essence what these terms mean depends on the circumstances in which they are being applied.

For example, it is only reasonable to expect that there will be suitable and sufficient lighting to ensure effective cleaning or food preparation to be undertaken safely and diligently.

**Q221 Surely ISO 9000, the quality standard, would assist environmental health departments throughout the UK to achieve a more uniform inspection standard?**

A Certainly this is one route to the pursuit of quality which many local authorities are either in the process of undertaking or are considering. ISO 9000 describes a uniformity rather than a quality. The Government is doing much to ensure uniformity by other means which have been addressed in other questions.

**Q222 If butchers' shops now have to be licensed what are the future implications for caterers who do extensive meat preparation?**

A There is probably more risk from catering activities which involve both cooked and raw products and therefore wider licensing is a possibility for the future. The licensing of butchers' shops is seen very much as a pilot and is being done as a result of the Lanarkshire E.coli 0157 food poisoning outbreak and the subsequent Pennington report on the Fatal Accident Enquiry. Should there be a similar incident in the catering world this will surely hasten the implementation of wider licensing.

**Q223 What does butchers' shop licensing depend on and is it a guarantee that my butcher is safe?**

A The three key criteria are:

- compliance with the **Food Safety (General Food Hygiene) Regulations 1995** with respect to the cleanliness, structure and food preparation conditions in the shop
- ensuring that staff are trained in food hygiene and there is a manager with specific training in hazard analysis
- ensuring that there is a HACCP system in place and operating.

In some ways it can be a guarantee of safety but regular enforcement by inspection EHOs will be necessary to ensure the standards are maintained.

**Q224 What are my legal obligations with respect to labelling menu items that contain peanuts?**

A There is no legal requirement, however there has been Department of Health advice that items should be properly identified. Service staff should be made aware through training so that they can inform customers should they require advice.

Generally, the small percentage of people that have a peanut allergy are aware of it and do all that they can to avoid peanuts. Chefs could do their bit by not putting peanuts in dishes that do not normally contain them.

**Q225 Why is there such a growth in the number of people affected by food allergies?**

A It is difficult to say and there are many schools of thought. Some health professionals believe we are becoming more sensitive to our "manufactured" environment and others suggest it is hereditary. There is an increasing use of more manufactured foods and food additives but there is a growing number of the population allergic to basic commodities: gluten, peanuts, milk products, etc. In reality it is still a small problem and should be put into context. However, more research is necessary in this important area of public health.

**Q226 How does the concept of "due diligence" under the Food Safety Act 1990 link with hazard analysis?**

A In court it is doubtful whether due diligence can be established as a defence against prosecution if hazard analysis has not been carried out and implemented. This is because many of the working procedures and record keeping at critical control points is the evidence needed to establish due diligence.

**Q227 I have been asked by my EHO to increase the mobility of my kitchen equipment, to assist cleaning. Can this be insisted upon and are there any options, given the cost of this?**

A This can be insisted on as Chapter V — Equipment of Schedule 1 of the **Food Safety (General Food Hygiene) Regulations 1995** provides for accessibility under and around equipment for cleaning. If you can ensure cleaning by another means, you may be able to negotiate a more cost-effective way forward. More advice is contained in the Industry Guide to Good Catering Practice obtainable from Chadwick House Group Publishing. Tel: 020 7928 6006.

# INDEX

## A



## B



## C

## G



## H



## I



## K



## L

## W



## Y